THE WHAT'S HAPPENING TO MY BODY?
BOOK FOR GIRLS

THE WHAT'S HAPPENING TO MY BODY? BOOK FOR GIRLS

A Growing Up Guide for Parents and Daughters

LYNDA MADARAS
with AREA MADARAS

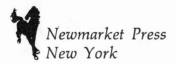
Newmarket Press
New York

0

Library of Congress Cataloging in Publication Data
Madaras, Lynda.
 What's happening to my body?

 Bibliography: p.
 Includes index.
 1. Adolescent girls—Growth.   2. Adolescent girls—
Health and hygiene.   3. Sex instruction for girls.
I. Madaras, Area.   II. Title.
RJ144.M3   1983   612'.661   83-8202
ISBN 0-937858-25-0
ISBN 0-937858-21-8 (pbk.)

Manufactured in the United States of America

Illustrations by Claudia Ziroli

My half of this book is dedicated to my present school, S.M.A.S.H. (Santa Monica Alternative School House), especially to Linda Gesualdi, my math teacher, Diana Garcia, my English teacher, and most of all, to my science teacher and advisor, Brian Lamagna (who I still insist is wrong, I won't take up writing as a profession). And this book is also dedicated to all the fathers of the world, since I don't believe they receive enough credit for the birth and upbringing of their children.—A.M.

For the students and staff at Sequoyah School, Pasadena, California.—L.M.

CONTENTS

LIST OF ILLUSTRATIONS

FOREWORD
by Ralph I. Lopez, M.D.

Back in 1969, as I finished my training in pediatrics, I saw a huge void in the delivery of health care for adolescents. A new field was rearing its subspecialty head, and the discipline of Adolescent Medicine began to formulate itself as falling somewhere between pediatrics and internal medicine, borrowing as well from its dermatologic, gynecologic, and psychiatric colleagues. Those of us who were interested in working with adolescents, from a medical point of view, were suddenly faced with the fact that there was very little medical literature directed to the care of the teenager. How to examine adolescents? How to deal with some of their questions? How to handle the extraordinary physical changes that were taking place? All of this had to be gathered from different sources. I remember vividly doing exactly what Ms. Madaras has done to gather information for her book. She also had to go to textbooks on gynecology, internal medicine, and pediatrics; she read the short paragraphs that pertained to this age group and compiled all that would be "readable" to the teenager.

It is now 1983 and recently much has been written on the medical care of the adolescent. In fact, no self-respecting pediatric text fails to include the word "adolescent" in its title. However, for the lay public (translation: all of my patients!) there still remained very little that they could read after lengthy explanations of the menstrual cycle or erections. Since my entire practice and all my lectures are geared to the teenager, this represented a huge deficiency in the process of teaching.

Many of the "this is your body" type of books are filled with complicated language and somehow seem to bypass the very audience they are trying to reach. When one talks about the fallopian tubes, or the cervical os, or premature ejaculations, it is difficult to imagine sustaining the interest of the sexually curious nine-, ten-, or eleven-year-old. But then, how many authors are willing to speak bluntly and frankly in such a way as to reach the target audience of the emerging adolescent?

Well, Lynda Madaras lays it on the line for both the kids and the parents. I have finally found a book that is clear and concise and that takes a no-holds-barred approach on so extraordinary a topic as your body. It is frank and may well offend some people who would prefer to keep youngsters in the dark ages about sexual information. Ms. Madaras deals with issues that involve sexuality in addition to the anatomy of sex. But I can guarantee you that if you can deal with the questions posed by the issues in this book when your child is a pre-teen, your relationship will be better when the turmoils of adolescence surface.

One of the wonderful aspects of this book is its insight into and candor about the roles and games that young girls play while emerging into womanhood. As a male—with a daughter whose one limitation has been that she can never be a father—I was intrigued as I peeked into a world that I had never experienced. In her introduction to the book, Ms. Madaras reveals the machinations of little-girl politics. For mothers this will serve as a reminder of their own youth and help with the turmoils of their daughters' world; for fathers it is a "must read" if they are to try to understand their daughters.

I enjoyed *The "What's Happening to My Body?" Book for Girls: A Growing Up Guide for Parents and Daughters.* To borrow a phrase from the commercial jingle, "If you're a grownup or plan to be one"—it's a great way to clear up a lot of misconceptions.

> RALPH I. LOPEZ, M.D.
> Director, Division of Adolescent Medicine
> The New York Hospital—Cornell Medical Center

FOREWORD
by Cynthia W. Cooke, M.D.

The "What's Happening to My Body?" Book for Girls takes a uniquely positive attitude toward the subject of female puberty. Throughout the ages male puberty has been greeted as a time of celebration—the arrival of manhood. Female puberty has often been closeted in shame, as if it were not at all the same process. There are centuries of tradition—both cultural and religious— that view the menstrual period as a time of uncleanliness or sickness. This negative attitude, coupled with the general resistance to sex education in the schools, has limited the availability of accurate information for young women until now.

Puberty and adolescence can be a devisive, traumatic time for many mother-daughter relationships. Recent explosions in sexual openness and explicitness in the media have broadened the communication gap between generations. Young women are beginning sexual activity at an earlier age, and though they seem to act in a more mature fashion than previous generations, they do not usually have a deep understanding of their bodies or psyches. They often act without considering the medical or social consequences.

As a gynecologist frequently confronted with such situations, I am delighted that this book, with its lucid and direct style, has been written. It provides an important starting ground for further discussion between mothers and daughters, and it will help set the direction for young women to keep informed, throughout their lives, about issues affecting their health.

CYNTHIA W. COOKE, M.D.
Clinical Assistant Professor, Obstetrics
and Gynecology, University of Pennsylvania
Co-author, *The Ms. Guide to a Woman's Health*

THE WHAT'S HAPPENING TO MY BODY?
BOOK FOR GIRLS

INTRODUCTION:
Why I Wrote This Book for My Daughter and Yours

It was one of those perfectly languid summer days when the heat is so rich and thick you can taste the scent of summer wildflowers in the air. My eight-year-old daughter and I were slowly making our way downstream through the woods by our house. It was one of those magic moments that sometimes happen between mothers and daughters. All the years of diaper changing, complicated child-care arrangements, hectic juggling of career and motherhood, nagging about bedrooms that need cleaning and pets that need feeding, all the inevitable resentments, conflicts, and quarrels seemed to fade away, leaving just the two of us, close and connected.

We stopped to sun ourselves on a rock, and my daughter shyly told me she had some new hairs growing on her body.

"Right down there," she pointed.

I was filled with pride as I watched her scrambling among the rocks, a young colt, long-limbed and elegant and very beautiful. I marveled at her assurance and ease. Her transition into womanhood would be so much more graceful than my own halting, jerky, and sometimes painful progress through puberty.

I was also proud of our relationship, proud that she felt comfortable enough to confide in me. Never in my wildest imaginings would I have thought of telling my mother that I'd discovered pubic hairs growing on my body. It was simply not something we could have discussed. I was glad that it was going to be different between my daughter and me.

3

We didn't talk much more about her discovery that day. Weeks and months passed without further mention of the topic, but our relationship remained close and easy.

"Enjoy it while you can," my friends with older daughters would tell me, "because once they hit puberty, it's all over. That's when they really get an attitude. There's just no talking to them." I listened in smug silence. I knew the stereotype: the sullen, sulky adolescent daughter and the nagging harpy of a mother who can't communicate with each other; but it was going to be different for us.

My daughter must have been nine or ten when it first started— her introduction to the nasty world of playground politics and the cruel games young girls play with each other. She'd arrive home from school in tears; her former best friend was now someone else's closest ally; she'd been excluded from the upcoming slumber party or was the victim of some other calculated schoolgirl snub. She'd cry her eyes out. I didn't know what to say.

"Well, if they're going to be like that, find someone else to play with," I'd say.

The tears flowed on. It got to be a weekly, then a twice-weekly event. It went on for months and months. And then I finally began to realize that no sooner than she had dried her tears, I would hear her on the telephone, maliciously gossiping about some other little girl, a former friend, and cementing a new friendship by plotting to exclude this other girl. I was indignant, and I began to point out the inconsistency in her behavior.

"You don't understand," she'd yell, stomping off to her bedroom and slamming the door.

She was right, I didn't understand. From time to time, I'd talk to the other mothers. It was the same with all of us. Why were our daughters acting like this? None of us had any answers.

"Well, girls will be girls," sighed one mother philosophically. "They all do it and we did the same when we were their age."

I reached back over the years, trying to remember. Were we really that horrible? Then I remembered The Powder Puffs, a club my girl friends and I belonged to. Unlike the Girl Scouts and the other adult-sanctioned after-school clubs, The Powder Puffs had no formal meetings, no ostensible purpose, which is not to say that the club didn't have a purpose. It did. The membership cards, which were wondrously official looking since one girl's father had run them off in his print shop, and which we carried around in the cloudy cellophane inserts of our identical vinyl, genuine leather wallets, certified us as members of the all-important Group. As if that weren't identification enough, we moved around in an inseparable herd, ate lunch together in our special territory of the playground, sat together giggling like a gaggle of geese in school assemblies, wrote each other's names on the canvas of our scuffed tennis shoes, combed our hair the same way, dressed alike, and generally made life miserable for the girls who were not members of our group.

Today, some twenty years later, I can only vaguely recall the names and faces of the other members of The Powder Puffs. I do, however, remember one girl so vividly that I can almost count the freckles on her face. Her name was Pam, and she was most emphatically not a member of the group, although she wanted desperately to be—so desperately, in fact, that she took to writing notes that she'd leave in my desk:

Dear Lynda,
Please, Please, Please let me join The Powder Puffs. If you say I'm OK, the rest of the girls will too. Please!!! Please!!!! Please!!!!! Please, please, please!
Pam

The notes embarrassed me horribly and, of course, the mere act of writing them doomed Pam forever to the status of outsider. I have conveniently forgotten how Pam fared after that. I know she never got to be a Powder Puff, and I imagine we made her life even more miserable with snickers and snubs, behind-the-back whisperings and the usual sorts of adolescent tactics. (I wonder if it would have been any comfort to Pam to have known that a year later, when my family moved to another state, I got my comeuppance. In the vulnerable position of "the new girl," I was the perfect target and boarded the school bus each day, pretending to be oblivious to the snickers and whispers that followed me up the aisle while I hunted for a seat.)

At any rate, what's really frightening is that I wasn't any more cruel than most adolescent girls. I talk to other women about their relationships with other girls during those years and hear the same sorts of stories. The milk of human kindness does not flow freely in the veins of pubescent girls.

We all remember how it was, and it was much the same for all of us. We had our best friend, from whom we were inseparable, with whom we shared our deepest secrets, and to whom we swore everlasting friendship. And then there was the larger gang, the other little girls at school. Everyone had a role: leader, follower, victim. Although the role assignments shifted from time to time, the roles themselves remained constant.

The games we played with each other were standardized as well and not very pretty. Exclusion was the basic format. One girl, for the crime of being the smartest, the prettiest, the ugliest, the dumbest, the most sexually developed, or whatever, was designated the victim. She was cast out, ostracized by the group.

But what was even more important, what was, in fact the central theme of my life in those years was a more personalized version of the exclusion game: betrayal by the best friend. In this case, the formerly inseparable friend was now unavailable for after-school activities, Saturday afternoon movies, and so forth. Her time was taken up with the new best friend. We were abandoned, crushed, and heartbroken; we cried our eyes out.

Little boys don't spend their energies in such melodramatic psychodramas. There's the gang or, more likely, the team, even the best friend and, undoubtedly, lots of exclusion, especially for the unathletic, quiet, and gentler boys, but there is not the same intensity in their interpersonal relationships nor the petty and vicious aspects that characterize the relationships between girls of this age.

Maybe, I thought, the mother who sighed that business about "girls being girls" was right. We all did it, and now it was happening all over again. Our daughters were playing the same games, by the same rules. Maybe it was inevitable. Maybe it was just the nature of the beast. I didn't like this idea, but there it was.

To add to the things I didn't like, there was a growing tension between my daughter and me. She was terribly moody, and it seemed as if she was always angry with me. And I was often angry with her. Of course, we'd always quarreled, but now the quarrels were almost constant. The volume of our communications reached a new decibel level. There was an ever-present strain between us.

All of this bothered me a great deal, but what was even more disturbing was the change in her attitude about her body. In contrast to the shy wonder that greeted her first pubic hairs, there was now a complete horror at the idea of developing breasts and having her first period. Like most "modern" mothers, I wanted my daughter's transition from childhood to womanhood to be a comfortable, even joyous, time. I had intended to provide her with all the necessary information in a frank, straightforward manner. This, or so went my reasoning, would eliminate any problems.

But, here was my daughter telling me she didn't want to grow breasts or have her first period. I asked why, but didn't get much further than "because I donwanna." I countered with an it's-great-to-grow-up pep talk that rang hollow even to my own ears.

Clearly something was amiss. I thought I'd made all the necessary information available in the most thoroughly modern manner, but the anticipated results, a healthy and positive attitude toward her body, had not materialized.

I thought long and hard about all of this, and finally I began to realize that I hadn't given my daughter all the information I thought I had. Although she was amazingly well informed about the most minute details of ovum and sperm, pregnancy and birth, the physical details of intercourse, and even the emotional content of love-making, she knew nothing, or next to nothing, about menstruation and the changes that would take place in her body over the next few years. She'd seen me in the bathroom changing a tampon, and I'd tossed off a quick explanation of menstrual periods, but I'd never really sat down and discussed the topic with her. I'd read her any number of marvelous children's books that explain conception, birth, and sexuality, but I'd never read her one about menstruation. Obviously, it was time to do that.

So, full of purpose, I trotted off to the library and discovered

that there was no such book.* There were one or two books for
young girls that briefly mentioned the topic, but they were
hopelessly out of date, and the tone was all wrong. Some of them
even made menstruation sound like a disease.

If I wanted to teach my daughter about menstruation and the
other changes that would happen in her body, I was obviously
going to have to rely on my own resources. Coincidentally, I
had just finished negotiating a contract to write a book on
women's health care. I would have to do considerable research
on menstruation for the book anyhow. (For once in my life, my
career as a writer and the job of being a mother wouldn't be
totally at loggerheads.)

The more deeply I researched the topic, the less surprised I
was that there was no book for young girls on menstruation.
Throughout history, in culture after culture, menstruation has
been a taboo subject. The taboo has taken many forms: One
must not eat the food cooked by a menstruating woman; touch
objects she has touched; look into her eyes; have sex with her.
We no longer believe that the glance of a menstruating woman
will wither a field of crops, that her touch will poison the water
in the well, that having sex with her will make a man's penis
fall off, but the menstrual taboo is, nonetheless, alive and well.

Even today, in an era when the most bizarre of incestual and
sado-masochistic sexual practices are the subject of cover stories
in national news magazines, cocktail chitchat, and television
specials, the natural bodily process of menstruation remains an
unmentionable subject. Indeed, as Paula Weidigger points out
in her excellent book *Menstruation and Menopause*, when the
subject of menstruation finally did come up on a segment of the
controversial TV show *All in the Family*, the network received
more letters protesting public mention of "such a thing" than
had been received as a result of the airing of any other segment
of the popular series (and this from a show that had dealt with
such topics as premarital sex, racial prejudice, impotency, and
homosexuality).

Of course, we are no longer banished to menstrual huts each

* Since that time, some excellent books have come out. See "For
Further Reading" in the back of this book.

month, as were our ancestral mothers in more primitive societies. But as Nancy Friday argues in *My Mother, My Self,* our release from monthly exile does not necessarily represent a more enlightened view of menstruation. Rather, Friday says, thanks to centuries of conditioning, we have so completely internalized the menstrual taboo that it's simply no necessary to bother any longer with menstrual huts. Our modern tribe needn't go to such lengths to remove any disturbing sight or mention of menstruation from its collective consciousness. We do it ourselves, through our ladylike avoidance of any public discussion of the topic and our meticulous toilet-paper mummification of our bloodied pads and tampons.

Indeed, we are so embarrassed by menstruation that we cannot even call it by its rightful name, relying instead on largely negative terms such as "the curse" or "falling off the roof." One male writer of a review of a book about menstruation, who Friday quotes, put it in a particularly telling perspective.

> If men menstruated they would probably find a way to brag about it. Most likely they would regard it as a spontaneous ejaculation, an excess of vital spirits. Their cup runneth over. Their sexuality supererogates. They would see themselves as "spending" blood in a plentitude of conspicuous waste. Blood, after all, is generally considered a good. "Blood" sports used to be the true test of manhood. And at the conclusion of a boy's first hunt he used to be "blooded." All that is turned around when it is the woman who bleeds. Bleeding is interpreted as a sign of infirmity, inferiority, uncleanliness and irrationality.*

It is certainly true that we don't often hear women boasting about their periods.

No "cup runneth over" for us, no solemn and magic puberty rites. Hardly anywhere in the anthropologies and histories of the kaleidoscope of cultures this planet has spawned are there

---

* Nancy Friday, *My Mother, My Self* (New York: Delacorte, 1977), pp. 147–48.

societies where women take their daughters out on moon-full nights to celebrate the ripening of the seeds of being we carry in our blood-lined bellies. There have rarely been joyous puberty rites for women. Instead, the years of puberty leading up to menarche, the first menstruation, are characterized by separation and conflict between mothers and daughters, and the whole topic is surrounded by a resounding silence.

So total is our silence that we ourselves are sometimes not aware of it.

"Oh, yes," the mother says, "I told my daughter all about it."

"My mother never told me anything," the daughter says.

Even if we are conscious of this silence and decide that it is time that this deplorable situation was dealt with, the taboos and our cultural embarrassment about menstruation may still take their toll. Wanting our daughters to have a positive view of their natural bodily functions, particularly if we have suffered in this area, we summon up our courage and carefully rehearse the proper lines. Intent upon improving the script our mothers wrote for us, we boldly announce to our daughters: "Menstruation Is a Wonderful Part of Being a Woman, a Unique Ability of Which You Should Be Proud."

At the same time, none of us would think of hiding our toothbrushes under the sink or in the back corners of the bathroom cupboard, yet it is rare to find a box of sanitary napkins prominently displayed next to the deodorants, toothpastes, and hair sprays that line the bathroom shelves of most homes. Thus, we constantly contradict our brave words and send our daughters double messages. We say it's fine and wonderful, but our unconscious actions indicate just the opposite. And, as we all know, actions speak louder than words.

The sad truth is that most of us have very little in the way of positive images to offer our daughters. Indeed, most of us are remarkably ignorant of even the basic facts about our bodies and our menstrual cycle.

"I'd hate to tell you how old I was before I learned that the Tampax I'd been inserting for years didn't enter the same passage through which I urinated," writes Nancy Friday.*

"My experience has been that seventy-five percent of the

---

* Friday, p. 137.

women in this country (and that's a modest estimate) couldn't give an explanation of menstrual periods to a sixth grader. They don't know how it happens, have little or no idea what does go on in their bodies," reports one health professional in Friday's book.*

As a result of the research I was doing, I was learning quite a bit about the physiological processes of menstruation. I could at least give a coherent explanation to a sixth grader, but I was also learning that I had a whole host of negative attitudes about menstruation in the back of my mind, attitudes that I had not even been conscious of before. These attitudes were changing, but who knew what else might be still lurking in the dark corridors of my subconscious? If I talked to my daughter about menstruation, I could say the right words, but would my body language, my tone of voice (and all those other unconscious ways of communicating) betray my intended message?

I worried about all of this for entirely too long a time, until the obvious solution sneaked up on me: I simply explained to my daughter that, when I was growing up, people thought of menstruation as something unclean and unmentionable. Now that I was older and more grown up, my attitudes were changing. But some of the feelings I had were old ones that I had lived with for a long time, all my life in fact, and they were hard to shake off. Sometimes they still got in my way without my even knowing it. This, of course, made perfect sense to my daughter, and from this starting point, we began to learn about our bodies together.

We didn't sit down and have The Talk. My mother sat me down one day to have The Talk, and I suppose she must have explained things in a comprehensive way, but all I remember was my mother being horribly nervous and saying a lot of things about babies and blood and that when It happened to me, I could go to the bottom drawer of her dresser and get some napkins. I wondered why she was keeping the napkins in a dresser drawer instead of in the kitchen cabinet where she usually kept them, but it didn't seem like a good time to ask questions.

Having one purposeful, nervous discussion didn't seem like it would fill the bill. Puberty is a complicated topic and it takes

* Friday, p. 137.

more than one talk. I decided just to keep the topic in mind and bring it up now and again. It turned out to be a pretty natural thing to do since I was doing so much research on the female body. In one of the medical texts I was plodding through, there was a section on puberty that discussed the five stages of pubic hair and breast development, complete with photos. I read the section to my daughter, translating from medicalese into English, so she would know when and how these changes would happen in her body.

I talked to her about what I was learning about the workings of the menstrual cycle. I showed her some magnificent pictures taken inside a woman's body at the very moment of ovulation as the delicate, fingerlike projections on the end of the fallopian tubes were reaching out to grasp the ripe egg.

A friend's mother gave us a wonderful collection of booklets from a sanitary napkin manufacturer that dated back over a period of thirty years. We read them together, laughing at the old-fashioned attitudes, attitudes I'd grown up with.

In the course of our reading, we learned that most girls begin to have a slight vaginal discharge a year or two prior to menstruation. I had told my daughter that when she started to menstruate, I would give her the opal ring that I always wore on my left hand, and that she, in turn, could pass it on to her daughter one day. But when she discovered the first signs of vaginal discharge, we were both so elated that I gave her the opal ring on the spot. (She'll get a matching one when she has her first menstrual period.)

A few hours later, as I sat working at my typewriter, I heard my daughter yelling to me from the bathroom, "Hey, Mom, guess what I got twenty-one of?"

We had a pregnant cat at the time and, for a few horrible moments, I was struck numb with the thought of twenty-one kittens. But, it wasn't kittens. My daughter was back to counting pubic hairs.

The time that we'd spent learning about menstruation and puberty had paid off. My daughter had regained her sense of excitement about the changes that were taking place in her body. This healthy attitude toward her body alone made our discussions worthwhile, but there were also other changes. First of all, things between the two of us got much better. We were back to our old, easy footing. She didn't magically start cleaning her bedroom or anything like that. We still had our quarrels, but they subsided to a livable level. And when we fought, at least we were fighting about the things we said we were fighting about. The underlying resentment and tension that had been erupting from beneath even our mildest disagreements, engulfing us in volcanic arguments, was gone.

But the most amazing change, perhaps because it was so unexpected, was that my daughter's role in the playground machinations had begun to change. In *My Mother, My Self*, Friday suggests the mother's failure to deal with her daughter's dawning sexuality, her silence about menstruation and the changes in the daughter's body, is perceived by the daughter as a rejection of the daughter's feminine and sexual self.

This silent rejection of these essential elements of self, coming as it does just at the time in the daughter's life when these very aspects of femininity and sexuality are manifesting themselves in the physical changes of her body, is nothing short of devastating. The daughter feels an overwhelming sense of rejection from the figure in her life with whom she is most intensely identified. One of the ways in which the daughter seeks to cope, to gain some control over her emotional life, is through the psychodramas of rejection that she continually reenacts with her peers.

I don't know if all this is true, but when I read Friday's book, I was reminded of a psychology experiment I'd seen in college. Rats in this experiment would press a lever and give themselves a jolting electric shock rather than receive random, intermittent shocks at the erratic whim of the experimenter. Self-administered shocks, even if they are more frequent and more intense, are apparently preferable to the anxiety of awaiting the unexpected, over which there is no control. Perhaps for little girls this small element of control, these self-administered rejections, are also attempts at reducing anxiety.

Or perhaps these dramas of rejection are more along the lines of the pecking-order behavior we see among chickens.

The largest, boldest chicken pecks another smaller one away from the feed dish, that chicken retaliates by pecking on another smaller and more vulnerable chicken, and so on down the line. We cannot deal with mother's rejection directly by confronting her. We are too small, too vulnerable, too defenseless; so, in a classic case of displaced aggression, we turn around and attack another little girl. Or perhaps just the opportunity to act out rejection, whether we play the role of leader, follower, or victim, to make this devastating experience familiar, to carve out roles we at least know and are used to, provides some measure of relief.

Whatever the particular mechanism, I can't help but suspect that the cultural taboo about menstruation, a mother's ignorance of and reluctance to deal with the topic, and the phenomena of playground politics are inextricably tied up with one another.

One morning, sometime after my daughter and I had begun to return to our old footing, I was driving her to school when she started to talk about the problems she was having with her friends. I held my breath. This topic had become so volatile that I hadn't even broached it in months. I didn't want to say the wrong thing.

"I don't know what to do, Mommy," she told me. "I want to be Susan's and Tanya's friend, but they're always whispering and talking about Kathy, and they do it loud enough so she can hear. And I'm with them, but I really like Kathy too."

"Well, can't you be friends with everybody?" I said, biting my tongue almost as soon as I said it. This had been one of my stock replies whenever we had talked about the subject, and it usually caused a storm, but this time she merely answered me, "But if I don't get down on Kathy with them, Susan and Tanya won't be friends with me."

"So what do you do when that happens; how do you handle it?" I asked, trying to say something neutral.

"Well, I just kind of stand there. I don't actually say bad things about Kathy, but I'm there with Susan and Tanya, so it's like I'm against Kathy too. And it makes me feel terrible, like I'm not a very good person," she said, starting to cry. "I don't know what to do."

"Well, look," I said, "Susan and Tanya are both really nice girls. Why don't you just go up to them and say 'Look, I have a problem and it's really making me feel lousy,' and then just tell them what you told me—that you want to be their friend, but you don't dislike Kathy and it makes you feel lousy if you join in putting her down."

My daughter gave me a look that told me what she thought of my suggestion.

"Not such a good idea, huh?" I offered.

"No, Mom," she agreed, and I kissed her goodbye as the school bell rang. Maybe my advice wasn't much help. Maybe it wasn't even very good advice, but at least we'd talked about the subject with each other.

Two days later, when I picked her up from school, she told me, "Well, I tried doing what you said to do."

"How did it work?"

"It worked. Susan and Tanya said that it was okay, that they'd still be friends with me even if I didn't hate Kathy."

Big of them, I thought to myself, but I didn't say anything. In truth, I was pleased; my daughter had begun to carve out a new role in the game for herself.

Perhaps Nancy Friday was right. Maybe my daughter perceived my attention to the changes taking place in her body as an acceptance of her sexual self, and this, in turn, lessened her need to participate in these playground psychodramas of rejection. I didn't, and still don't, know whether Friday's theories are real explanations, but my experiences with my own daughter certainly seemed to validate her ideas. Still, I wouldn't want to go so far as to promise you that spending time teaching your daughter about menstruation and the other physical changes of puberty will magically deliver her from the psychodramatics of puberty or will automatically erase the tensions that so often exist between parents and their adolescent daughters. But my experiences with my own daughter and, more recently, as the teacher of a class on puberty and sexuality for teens and pre-teens, have convinced me that kids of this age need and want information about what is happening to them at this point in their lives.

This information isn't always easy to come by. Too often we parents simply don't have the facts to give our children. Most of us have, at best, a sketchy knowledge of menstruation, and it is a rare parent who can describe the five stages of breast or pubic hair development. This book was written to provide those facts.

The book is designed to be read by girls in the nine- to thirteen-year-old age group, but may also be appropriate for younger or older girls. It details the physiological changes in the female body during puberty. This book does not pretend to cover all the things you will need to discuss with your daughter as she goes through puberty. What book could? It is only a beginning. For example, it doesn't go into detail on topics like birth control, venereal disease, rape, abortion, drugs, the changing relationship between parent and child, or with making decisions about sexual intercourse—not because I don't think these topics should be discussed with kids of this age. On the contrary, I think it's very important to do so, but there are already many excellent books that deal specifically with these topics. Some are suggested in "For Further Reading" at the end of this book.

This book, and those I mention in the bibliography, may reflect values that are not the same as yours. This doesn't mean that you can't use them. You don't have to throw out the baby with the bathwater. Instead, you can use these books as an opportunity to explain your own point of view. For example, the topic of masturbation comes up in Chapter 5 of this book. The discussion of masturbation reflects my attitude—that masturbation is a perfectly fine, perfectly healthy thing to do. This attitude may conflict with your moral or religious views. If that's the case, you can read this section with your child, explaining how and why you feel the way you do.

Ideally, this book is something that you and your daughter will come back to time and time again as she progresses through puberty. You may want to introduce her to the book when she is eight or nine, before these changes have started to happen, so she'll have some idea of what to expect. But do come back to it again when she is actually going through them. What she is able to absorb when she is eight or nine will be much different from what she is able to absorb a couple of years later.

I hope that this book will help you and your daughter understand the changes that take place in a girl's body during puberty, and that by reading it together, the two of you will become that much closer and more comfortable with each other.

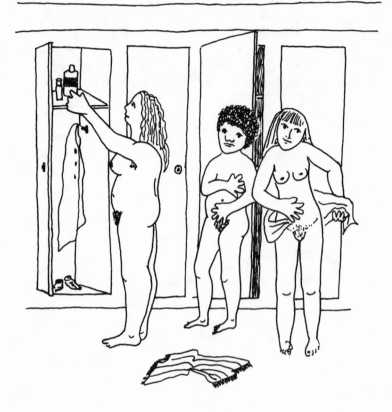

CHAPTER 1

Puberty

This book is about a time in a girl's life when her body is changing from a child's body into a woman's body. This time of changing is called puberty.

As you can see from the drawing facing this page, our bodies change quite a bit as we go through puberty. We get taller. The general shape or contour of our bodies changes: Our hips and thighs get fleshier, and we take on a more rounded, curvy shape. Our breasts begin to swell and to blossom out from our chests. Soft nests of hair begin to grow under our arms

puberty (PEW-bur-tee)   The word *puberty* is pronounced with the accent on the first part of the word, PEW. You say that part of the word with the most emphasis. Throughout this book, there are a number of words that you may not have heard before. Whenever we use these words for the first time, we will include a pronunciation key like this at the bottom of the page.

and in the area between our legs. Our skins begin to make new oils that change the very feel and smell of us. At the same time that these changes are happening on the outside, other changes are taking place inside our bodies.

These changes don't happen overnight. Puberty happens slowly and gradually, over a period of many months or years. These changes may start when a girl is as young as eight, or they may not begin until she is sixteen or older. Regardless of when they start for you, you'll probably have a lot of questions about what is happening to your body. We hope that this book will answer at least some of these questions.

"We" are my daughter, Area, and I. The two of us worked together to make this book. We talked to doctors and research scientists and pored over medical textbooks. We also talked to mothers and daughters, to find out what happened to them during puberty, how they felt about it, and what kinds of questions they had. You'll hear their voices throughout this book. Some of the quotes in this book are from kids in my class. During the school year, I teach a class on puberty once a week at Sequoyah School in Pasadena, California. (My daughter used to go to Sequoyah, which is how I happen to be teaching there.) The kids in my class and the mothers and daughters we talked with had a lot of questions and a lot of things to say about puberty. So, in a sense, they too helped write the book.

I usually start the first puberty class of the year by talking about how babies are made. This seems like a good place to begin since the changes that occur during puberty happen to get the body ready for a time in our lives when we may decide to have a baby.

A talk with a group of boys and girls about how babies are made usually turns into a pretty giggly affair, because in order to talk about how babies are made, we have to talk about *sex*, and sex, as you may have noticed, is a *very big deal*. People often act embarrassed, secretive, giggly, or some other strange way when the topic of sex comes up.

Even the word itself is confusing, because *sex* can mean many different things and is used in different ways. In the simplest meaning of the word, *sex* refers to the different kinds of bodies that men and women have. There are a number of differences between male and female bodies, but the most obvious is that a male has a penis and scrotum and a female has a vulva and vagina. These body parts, or organs, are called *sex organs*. People are either members of the male sex or the female sex, depending on which type of sex organs they have.

The word *sex* is also used in other ways. We may say that two people are "having sex." Having sex, or sexual intercourse, involves a man putting his penis into a woman's vagina. Or we may say that two people are "being sexual with each other," which means that they are having sexual intercourse or that they are holding, touching, or caressing each other's sex organs. We may also say that we are "feeling sexual," which means that we are having feelings or thoughts about our sexual organs, about being sexual with another person, or about having intercourse.

Our sexual organs are very private parts of our bodies. We usually keep them covered up, and we don't talk about them in public very often. Having sex, being

penis (PEE-niss)
scrotum (SKRO-tum)
vulva (VUL-va)
vagina (vah-JIE-nah)
intercourse (IN-ter-korse)

sexual with someone, or having sexual feelings are also usually private matters that don't get talked about very often. So when I come into a classroom and start talking about penises and vaginas and having sex . . . well, things get pretty giggly. (You can imagine how my poor daughter felt, having her mother coming to school to talk about *those* things. Before I started teaching the class, I asked her if it was okay with her. She wasn't entirely happy with the idea. Finally she said all right, but no way was she going to be in the class! As it turned out, the classes were a big hit. Kids were coming up to her and saying how much they liked the class. So eventually she joined the class too, even though she'd heard most of this stuff at home.)

I decided that if we were going to get all silly and giggly in class when we talked about these things, we might as well get *really* silly and giggly. So, I start the first class of the year by giving everyone photocopies of the two drawings in Illustration 1 and red and blue colored pencils that we use to color the drawings.

Sex Organs

Illustration 1 shows the male and the female sex organs. These sex organs are also referred to as the *genitals*, or the *genital organs*. Everyone has sex organs on both the inside and the outside of the body, and they change as you go through puberty. These pictures show how the sex organs on the outside of the body look in grown men and women.

I generally begin with the male sex organs. I explain that the sex organs on the outside of a man's body have two main parts and that the scientific names for these parts are the *penis* and the *scrotum*. By the

genitals (JEN-a-tulls)

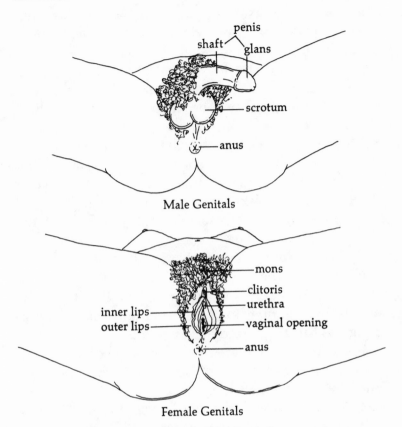

Male Genitals

Female Genitals

Illustration 1. The Genitals

time I've passed out the copies of the drawings and have started talking about the penis and the scrotum, the kids in my classes are usually giggling like mad, nudging each other, or falling off their chairs in embarrassment. I don't pay too much attention to how they're acting, I just say, "Okay, the penis itself also has two parts: the shaft and the glans. Find the shaft of the penis on your drawing and color it blue." Some kids keep giggling and some get very intent, but they all

glans (GLANZ)

start coloring. Why don't you color the shaft too (unless, of course, this book belongs to someone else or to a library. One of the people we admire most in the world is a wonderful lady named Lou Ann Sobieski. She's a librarian, and my daughter and I would be in very hot water if Lou Ann thought we were telling people to color on library books.)

Moving right along—the glans of the penis has a ridge of skin around it called the *corona*, and after they've colored the shaft blue, I tell my class to color the corona red. Next, we color in the glans itself. I usually recommend blue and red stripes, but color it any way you want, just as long as it's colored differently from the other parts so that it will stand out clearly.

Next comes the scrotum. "Red and blue polka dots for the scrotum," I tell my class. By this time, the picture is beginning to look rather silly, and the giggling has turned to outright laughter.

Inside the scrotum are two egg-shaped organs called *testes*, or *testicles*. You can't see them in these pictures, but I like to mention them at this point because they have a lot to do with making babies. We'll talk more about them in the following pages.

Finally, I ask my class to color the anus. The anus is the opening through which feces or bowel movements leave our bodies. It is not really a sex organ, but since it is located in the genital area, I like to mention it.

The business of coloring in the different parts like this works well because it gets everyone laughing and

corona (ko-RO-na)
testes (TES-teez)
testicles (TES-ti-kuls)
anus (AY-nus)
feces (FEE-sees)
bowel (BOW-ul)

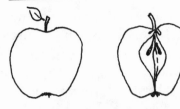

If you cut an apple in half, you would be able to see the seeds and core on the inside of the apple. This drawing, which shows the inside of an apple, is called a cross section.

The drawing below is also a cross section. It shows the inside of the penis and scrotum.

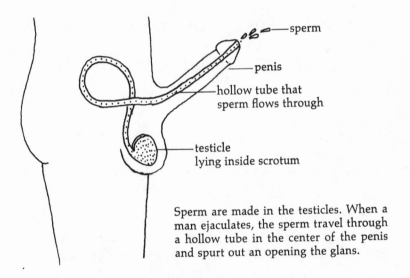

Sperm are made in the testicles. When a man ejaculates, the sperm travel through a hollow tube in the center of the penis and spurt out an opening the glans.

Illustration 2. Cross Section of the Penis and Scrotum

makes it easier to deal with the nervousness many of us feel when we talk about sex organs. But I also have the kids do it for another reason: I think it helps them to learn the names of these organs. If you just look at the drawing and see that this part is labeled *penis* and that part *scrotum*, it's all kind of jumbled and doesn't stick in your mind. But if you spend a few moments coloring them in, you have to pay attention and you'll remember better. These are important parts of the body, so it's worth the effort. If this book isn't yours and you can't color in it, try making a tracing of these drawings and coloring on the tracings.

While everyone in my class is busy coloring pictures, we talk about slang words. People don't always use the scientific names for these body parts. The kids in our classes came up with quite a list of slang words for the penis, scrotum, and testicles.

SLANG WORDS FOR THE PENIS, SCROTUM, AND TESTICLES

PENIS		SCROTUM AND TESTICLES
cock	peter	balls
dick	rod	nuts
prick	dingus	eggs
schlong	dork	rocks
wee-wee	meat	jewels
wanger	pisser	cubes
pecker	hot dog	bags

Personally, I don't object to slang words, but some people do, and they may get upset if they hear you using them. You may or may not care about upsetting people in this way, but you should at least be aware of the fact that there are people who find slang words offensive.

When we've finished coloring the male sex organs, we move on to the female sex organs. The genital organs on the outside of a woman's body are sometimes referred to as the *vulva.* The vulva has many parts. We usually start at the top with the fleshy mound called the *mons* and color it with blue polka dots. Then we move toward the bottom of the mons

mons (MONZ)

where it divides into two folds or flaps of skin called the *outer lips*. Try coloring them with red stripes. In between the outer lips lie the inner lips. Try blue stripes for the inner lips. The inner lips join together at the top, and there is a small, bud-shaped organ called the *clitoris*. Color it red. Just down from the clitoris, between the inner lips, is the urinary opening, the opening through which urine (pee) leaves the body. Color it blue. Below the urinary opening is another opening called the vaginal opening. It leads into the hollow pouch or cavity on the inside of our bodies called the *vagina*. Use your imagination—color the vaginal opening red, blue, striped, or whatever. Finally, we come to the anus; choose a color and color the anus.

While we're coloring in the female genitals, we also make a list of slang words used to refer to this part of a woman's body.

SLANG WORDS FOR THE VULVA AND VAGINA

cunt	muff	beaver	snatch
pussy	stuff	honeypot	poontang
	box	hole	

By the time we've finished coloring both these pictures, everyone has giggled off a good deal of their embarrassment. They have also gotten a pretty good idea of where these body parts are, which makes it a lot easier to understand how a man and a woman make babies.

clitoris (KLIT-or-iss)
urinary (YUR-rin-air-ee)
urine (YUR-in)
vaginal (VAH-jin-ul)

Sexual Intercourse

When I tell the kids in my class what *sexual intercourse* means, they usually have two reactions. One is that they want to know just how a man's penis could get into a woman's vagina. I explain that sometimes the penis gets stiff and hard and stands out from the body. This is called an *erection,* and it can happen when a male is feeling sexual or is having sex with someone, and at other times too. (We'll say more about this later in the chapter "Puberty in Boys.") An erection happens because the spongy tissue inside the penis fills up with blood. Some people call an erection a "boner" or a "hard-on" because the penis feels so stiff and hard during an erection. It's almost as if there really is a bone in there. But there isn't any bone, just blood-filled, spongy tissue.

While it is erect, the penis can slide right into the vaginal opening. The vagina isn't very large, but it's very elastic and stretchy, so the erect penis can easily fit in there.

In addition to wanting to know *how,* some of the kids in our classes want to know *why* anyone would want to do this.

People have sexual intercourse for all sorts of reasons. It is a special way of being close with another person. It also feels good, which some of the kids in my class find hard to believe. But these areas of our bodies have many nerve endings; if they are stroked or rubbed in the right ways, these nerve endings send messages to pleasure centers in our brains. When our pleasure centers are stimulated, we get pleasurable feelings all over our bodies. People also have sexual

erection (e-REK-shun)

intercourse because they want to have a baby, but babies don't start to grow every time a man and woman have intercourse, just sometimes.

Making Babies

In order to make a baby, two things are needed: a seed from a woman's body, which is called an *ovum*, and a seed from a man's body, which is called a *sperm*.

Sperm are made inside the testicles, the two egg-shaped organs inside the scrotum. Sometimes, when a man and a woman are having sexual intercourse, the man ejaculates. When a man ejaculates, the muscles of his penis contract, and the sperm are pumped out of the testicles, through a hollow tube in the center of the penis, and spurt out an opening in the center of the glans, as shown in Illustration 2. A couple of spoonfuls of a creamy, white liquid, full of millions of tiny, microscopic sperm come out of the penis. This liquid is called "ejaculate," or in slang terms "come" or "jism."

After the sperm leave the penis, they start swimming up toward the top of the vagina. They pass through a tiny opening at the top of the vagina that leads into an organ called the *uterus* (see Illustration 3). The uterus is a hollow organ and, in a grown woman, it's only about the size of a clenched fist. But the thick, muscle walls of the uterus are quite elastic and, like a balloon, the uterus can expand to many times its size. The uterus has to be able to expand because it is here, inside a woman's uterus, that a baby grows.

ovum (OH-vum)
sperm (SPURM)
ejaculates (e-JACK-u-lates)
uterus (YOU-ter-us)

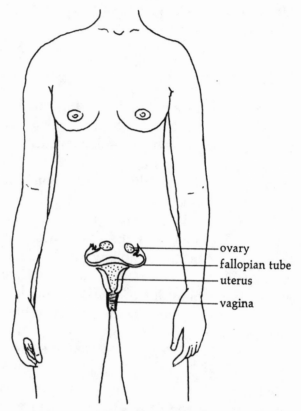

Illustration 3. The Sex Organs on the Inside of a Woman's Body

Some of the sperm swim up to the top of the uterus and into one of two little tubes, or tunnels, called the *fallopian tubes*. Not all the sperm make it this far. Some drift back down the uterus and out into the vagina where they join other sperm that never made it out of the vagina. These sperm and the rest of the creamy white liquid dribble back down the vagina and out of the woman's body.

fallopian (fuh-LOPE-e-an)

Women, too, make seeds in their bodies. When we are talking about just one of these seeds we use the word *ovum*. When we are talking about more than one, we use the word *ova*. The ova ripen inside two little organs called *ovaries*. In a grown woman, the ovaries produce a ripe seed about once a month. When this seed is ripe, it leaves the ovary and travels down the fallopian tube toward the uterus. If a woman and man have sexual intercourse around the time of the month when the ripe ovum has just left the ovary, there's a good chance that the sperm and ovum will meet inside the tube. When a sperm and ovum meet, the sperm penetrates the outer shell of the ovum and moves inside it. This joining together of the ovum and the sperm is called *fertilization*, and when a sperm has penetrated an ovum, the ovum has been fertilized.

Most of the time, the ovum travels through the fallopian tube without meeting up with a sperm, and the tiny ovum just disintegrates. But, if the ovum has been fertilized, it doesn't disintegrate. Instead, the fertilized seed plants itself on one of the inside walls of the uterus, and over the next nine months, it grows into a baby (see Illustration 4).

Menstruation

The inside walls of the uterus are covered by a special lining. Each month, as the ovum is ripening in the ovary, this lining gets ready just in case the ovum is going to be fertilized. The lining gets thicker. It also develops new blood passageways, for if the fertilized seed plants itself in the lining, it will need plenty of rich

ova (OH-vah)
ovaries (OH-vah-reez)

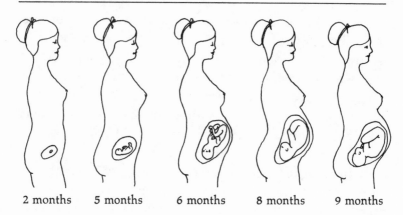

| 2 months | 5 months | 6 months | 8 months | 9 months |

Illustration 4. Stages of Pregnancy. A fertilized ovum plants itself on the inside wall of the uterus, and over the next nine months, it develops into a baby.

blood in order to grow and develop into a baby. Spongy tissues develop around these new blood passageways to cushion them. These tissues fill with blood and begin to make nourishment to help the seed to grow.

If the ovum is not fertilized by meeting a sperm in the tube, then this newly grown lining in the uterus will not be needed. So, about a week after the unfertilized ovum has disintegrated, the uterus begins to shed this lining. The spongy, blood-filled tissue of the lining breaks down and falls off the wall. It collects in the bottom of the uterus and dribbles out into the vagina. It then flows down the length of the vagina and out the vaginal opening (see Illustration 5).

This breaking down and shedding of the lining inside the uterus is called *menstruation*. When the bloody lining dribbles out of the vaginal opening, a woman is menstruating or, as we say, having her period.

menstruation (mens-stroo-AY-shun)
menstruating (mens-stroo-AY-ting)

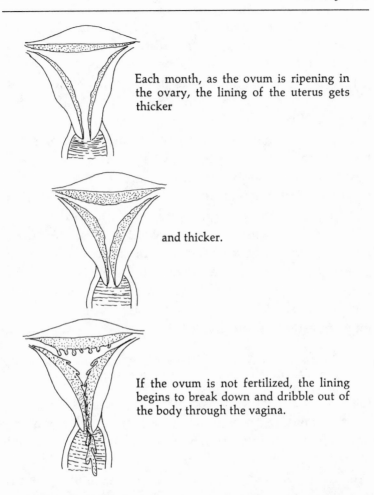

Each month, as the ovum is ripening in the ovary, the lining of the uterus gets thicker

and thicker.

If the ovum is not fertilized, the lining begins to break down and dribble out of the body through the vagina.

Illustration 5. Cross Section of the Uterus. The shaded area is lining of the uterus.

The amount of blood that dribbles out during a period varies. Some of us have a couple of tablespoons, others have almost a cupful. The blood doesn't come out all at once, but dribbles out slowly over a number of days. Then it stops. It may only take a couple of days or it may take a week or so for all of the menstrual blood to empty out of your body.

Once the bleeding has stopped, the uterus starts growing a new lining in preparation for next month's ripe ovum. If that ovum is not fertilized, the newly grown lining will again break down, and you will have another period, usually within a month or so after your last period.

A girl may have her first period any time between her eighth and sixteenth birthdays. A few girls will have their first period when they are younger or older than this, but the majority of the girls have their first period between their eighth and sixteenth birthdays.

In the following chapters, we'll talk more about menstruation, about having your first period, and about the other changes that will take place in your body as you grow older and go through puberty. If you're like the kids in my class, you'll probably have a lot of questions about these things.

Everything You Ever Wanted to Know . . .

It isn't always easy to ask certain questions. We may feel too embarrassed to ask or we may feel our questions are just too dumb. If you feel like that, you're not alone. In my classes, we play a game called "Everything You Ever Wanted to Know About Sex and Puberty, but Were Afraid to Ask." I pass out slips of paper at the beginning of each class so the kids can write down their questions and put them in a question box. They don't have to sign their names to the questions, and I'm the only one who gets to see them, so nobody can look at the handwriting and figure out who wrote the question. I also leave the locked box in place where people can get to it during the week in case they think up questions after class. At the end of each class, I take the questions out of the box, read them out loud, and answer them the best I can.

In writing this book, we've tried to answer all the questions that have come up in our "Everything You Ever Wanted to Know" game, but you may find that you have questions that aren't answered by this book. If so, perhaps your mom or dad, the school nurse, one of your teachers, or another adult can help you find answers to your questions. Or you could write to us. We'd love to hear about any questions or confusions you may have or about things you liked or didn't like about this book. Your envelope should be addressed like this:

Lynda and Area Madaras
Newmarket Press
3 East 48th Street
New York, New York 10017

Be sure to include your name and address so we can write back to you.

Using This Book

You may want to read this book with your parents, with a friend, or all by yourself. You may want to read it straight through from beginning to end, or you may want to jump around, reading a chapter here and there, depending on what you are most curious about. However you decide to go about reading this book, we hope that you'll enjoy it and that you'll learn as much from reading it as we did from writing it.

CHAPTER 2

Changing Size and Shape

If you notice that the jeans you bought just a couple of months ago are up around your ankles already or that your brand-new shoes are suddenly too small, it's probably because you are beginning to go through puberty. As you begin puberty, your body starts to grow at a faster rate.

The Growth Spurt

The sudden increase in the rate of growth at the start of puberty is called a "growth spurt." It happens at different ages for different girls, and is more noticeable in some girls than in others. It usually starts before you begin to develop breasts or to grow soft nests of hair in the area between your legs.

Starting around the age of two, the average girl grows about two inches a year until she starts puberty. When puberty begins, she may start growing twice as fast, so that she grows four inches that year instead of only two. Of course, not everyone is average, so you may grow more or less than this.

The growth spurt usually lasts less than a year, then the growth rate begins to slow down again. By the time you've had your first menstrual period, your growth rate has usually slowed back down to one or two inches a year. Most girls reach their full adult height within one to three years after their first period.

Boys go through a growth spurt during puberty too, but they usually don't start puberty until a couple of years after girls start. This is why eleven- and twelve-year-old girls are often taller than the boys their age. However, a couple of years later, when the boys start their growth spurt, they catch up to the girls and surpass them in height. Of course, some girls, the ones who are on the tall side, will always be taller than most of the boys. But often a girl who is taller than the boys she knows when she is eleven or twelve will find that the boys have caught up by the age of thirteen or fourteen.

During puberty, as you are growing taller, your bones are, of course, getting longer, but not all the bones in your body grow at the same rate. Your arms and legs tend to grow faster than your backbone during puberty, so you may notice that your arms and legs are longer in proportion to the trunk of your body than they were during childhood or than they will be when you reach adulthood.

The bones in your feet also grow faster than your other bones. Thus, your feet reach their adult size long before you've reached your adult height. A number of the girls we talked to worried about this. As one girl explained:

> I was just a little over five feet tall when I was eleven, but I wore a size eight shoe. I thought, Oh, no, if my feet keep on growing, they're gonna be gigantic! But I'm sixteen now, and I'm five feet eight inches tall, but my feet are still size eight.

In reaction to this, another girl said:

> I'm sure glad to hear that. I wear a size eight and a half now and I'm only twelve years old and five foot one and a half. People are always teasing me about my big feet. The last time I got tennis shoes, the guy in the store made some big joke about how if my feet got any bigger, he'd have to sell me the shoe boxes to wear. I pretended to laugh, but I was embarrassed and worried that maybe my feet were just going to keep getting bigger and bigger.

Changing Contours

As you go through puberty, your face changes. The lower part of your face lengthens and your face gets fuller. The general shape or contour of your body also changes. Your hips get wider as fat tissue grows around the hips, buttocks, and thighs so your body begins to have a rounder, curvier shape (see Illustration 6). Your breasts are also developing fat tissue, so they too get rounder and fuller. (We'll talk more about breasts in Chapter 4.)

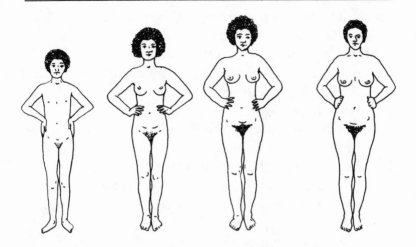

Illustration 6. Girls in Puberty. As we go through puberty, our hips get wider. Fat tissue begins to grow around our hips, thighs, and buttocks, giving our bodies a curvier shape. Our breasts begin to swell, and soft nests of hair begin to grow under our arms and on our genitals.

Liking Your Own Shape

Bodies come in all sorts of shapes and sizes—short or tall, thin or plump, narrow or wide, angular or curvy, straight or rounded. To some extent, you can change the shape of your body by diet and exercise. If you are thin, you can put on weight. If you are fat, you can diet so that your body loses some of its fat tissue. You can exercise to build up or slim down areas of your body. But you do have a basic shape to your body that can't be changed, no matter how much or how little you eat or what kind of exercise you do.

If you aren't satisfied with your body and are under- or overweight, perhaps you need to see a doctor and get on a diet and exercise plan to help you gain or lose weight. If you are not sure whether you're under- or overweight, your doctor can help you decide if your weight is within normal ranges for your height and body build. If you fall within these weight ranges and still aren't happy with the way your body looks, maybe you need to think about where you've gotten these ideas about how your body *should* look that are making you feel dissatisfied with the way you do look.

It would be nice if we could all just look at our bodies without having to compare them to someone else's and just say, "Hey, I like the way I look." But we live in a society where there's a lot of competition between people, between companies, and even between countries. We are always comparing and competing to see who's best. But who decides what's best?

Most of us get our ideas about what's the "best" or "most attractive" kind of female body from the pictures we see in magazines and billboards and from television and movies. Right now, in our country, these pictures usually show tall, thin, blond, blue-eyed, white-skinned women with rosy cheeks, no pimples or freckles, flat stomachs, tiny waists, long legs, big breasts, hairless legs and underarms, curvy hips and thighs—without a single bulge anywhere. As you may have noticed, there are few of us who actually look like this. For one thing, we aren't all white-skinned, blond-haired, and blue-eyed. And we aren't all thin with tiny waists and big breasts. We come in a pleasing array of sizes, shapes, and colors.

But when we are constantly bombarded with pictures of these glamorous images of skinny, blond, blue-eyed women, it can make us feel that there is something about our hips, breasts, thighs, height, shapes, faces, skin, or hair that is somehow not right.

If we don't look like these women, we may be unhappy with the way we look. In fact, people in this country are often so unhappy about their looks that they spend millions and millions of dollars each year on hair dyes, makeup, fad diets, leg and underarm hair removers, tummy flatteners, breast developers, waist trimmers, and on and on. Some people even have operations to make their tummies flatter, their noses straighter, or their breasts a different size.

With all the images of these "perfect" women who seem to be having glamorous lives and no problems at all, it's easy to get to thinking that these kinds of bodies actually *are* better or more attractive (see Illustration 7). If you get to feeling that way sometimes, it might help you to remember these bodies only seem to be more desirable because they are in fashion in our particular culture at this particular time. Being in fashion doesn't make a mini-skirt "better" than a knee-length skirt, and being in fashion doesn't make one body type "better" than another.

It helps, too, to remember that fashions change and that they vary from culture to culture. The drawings you see in Illustration 8 show bodies that have been in fashion in other times and in other cultures. The first drawing is a flapper from America in the 1920s. During the 1920s in this country, curvy bodies and big breasts were definitely not in fashion. In fact, women with big breasts wrapped their breasts tightly, strapping them down, so that they wouldn't stick out. The second drawing shows a woman from Europe in the 1500s. Today she would be considered a bit chunky, but back then her type of body was the "best," "most attractive" kind of body a woman could have. The third drawing shows a Polynesian woman. She hardly matches our culture's standard of beauty, but in her culture, she'd

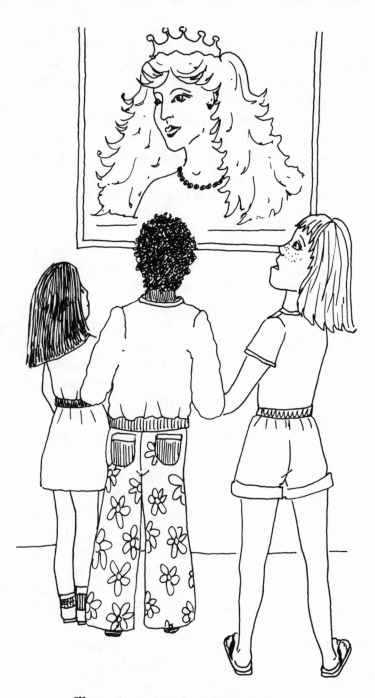

Illustration 7. Matching Cultural Ideals

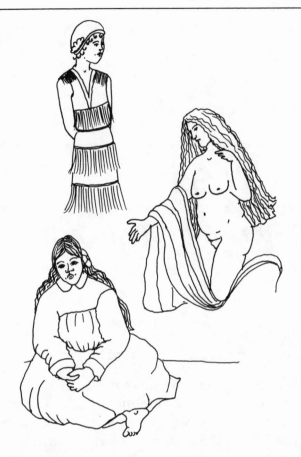

Illustration 8. Types of Beauty. From the top, clockwise, are a flapper, a woman from the 1500s, and a Polynesian woman.

be considered a great beauty and her rounded body would be considered the "best" and "most attractive."

Learning to appreciate yourself and to love your own body, regardless of whether or not it matches up with what's in fashion, is a big step in growing up. And if you can manage to find your own body attractive, other people will too, and it won't matter whether it's the so-called best or most attractive kind of body— not one bit. We guarantee it.

CHAPTER 3

Body Hair, Perspiration, and Pimples

For some girls, the growth spurt and the changes in the shape of their bodies are the first signs of puberty. For others, the first sign that puberty is beginning is that they start growing hair in new places on their bodies.

Pubic Hair

Pubic hair is the name given to the curly hairs that grow in the area of our bodies where our legs join together. This area has many names, such as the vulva or the genital area. Some people call this area of the body the vagina. Actually, the vagina is inside your body, so it is not really correct to call it the vagina.

pubic (PEW-bik)

If you stand sideways in front of a mirror, you'll notice that there is a little mound of flesh in this area that protrudes (sticks out) a bit. This mound is called the *mons*, which is a word from Latin that means little hill or mound. It is also called the *mons veneris*. *Veneris* is another Latin word that refers to Venus, the goddess of love, so *mons veneris* means "mound of Venus" or "mound of love." The mons is just one part of the vulva or genital area. We'll be talking about the other parts of the vulva later, but for now, let's concentrate on the mons.

The mons is a pad of fat tissue that lies under the skin. It cushions the pubic bone that lies beneath it. If you press down on the mons, you can feel the pubic bone underneath. For this reason, the mons is also referred to as the *pubis*. Regardless of what you call it, sooner or later you will begin to notice curly, colored hairs growing here.

If you look at your mons, you will notice that, toward the bottom, it divides into two folds or flaps of skin. These are the *labia majora*, or outer lips. In many girls, pubic hair first begins to grow on the edges of these lips. In others, it first begins growing on the mons itself.

Five Stages of Pubic Hair Growth

Doctors have divided pubic hair growth into the five different stages shown in Illustration 9. You may be in one of these stages or in between one stage and another. See if you can find the stage you're closest to.

veneris (ven-AIR-iss)
pubis (PEW-bis)
labia (LAY-bee-uh)
majora (may-JOR-ah)

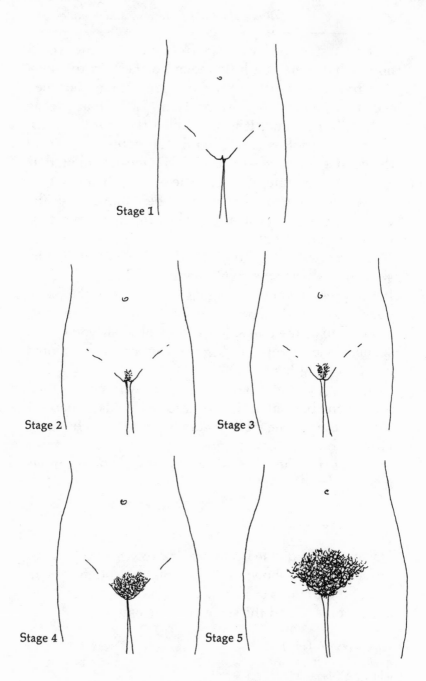

Stage 1

Stage 2

Stage 3

Stage 4

Stage 5

Illustration 9. The Five Stages of Pubic Hair Growth

Stage 1 starts when you are born and continues throughout childhood. In this stage the mons and the lips are either hairless or they have a few light-colored, soft hairs similar to the hair that may be growing on your belly. There aren't any pubic hairs.

Stage 2 starts when you grow your first pubic hairs. If you have hairs growing on your vulva during childhood, you will be able to tell the difference between these childhood hairs and pubic hairs because the pubic hairs are longer, darker in color, and curly. At first, they may be only slightly curly and there may be just a few of them. You may have to look very closely in order to see them.

In Stage 3, the pubic hairs get curlier and thicker, and there are more of them. They may get darker in color. They cover more of the mons and the lips than they did in Stage 2.

In Stage 4, the pubic hair gets still thicker and curlier, and it may continue to get darker in color. It also spreads out so it covers more of the mons and the lips.

Stage 5 is the adult stage. The pubic hair is thick and coarse and tightly curled. It covers a wider area than in Stage 4. It usually grows in an upside-down triangle pattern. In some women, the pubic hair grows up toward the belly button and out onto the thighs.

You may start growing pubic hair when you are only eight, or you may not start until you are sixteen or older. Most girls get to Stage 3 between the ages of eleven and thirteen. Most girls have their first menstrual period when they are in Stage 4, but many start their periods while they are still in Stage 3. A few will start their periods while they are only in Stage 2, and a few others won't start until after they've reached Stage 5. If you start your period while you are still in Stage 1 and your breasts haven't started to develop either, then you should see a doctor. Starting your period before you have any pubic hair and before your breasts have begun to develop doesn't necessarily mean that something is wrong, but it may mean that you have a problem. So you should see a doctor and get it checked out.

Color and Amount of Pubic Hair

Some women have lots of pubic hair, while on others, it is sparse. It may be blond, brown, black, or red and does not necessarily match the color of the hair on your head. The hair on your head may turn gray when you get old, and your pubic hair may also turn gray.

Why Pubic Hair?

One of the questions the girls in our class often ask is why we have pubic hair. Pubic hair helps keep the area between our outer lips clean. Just as our eyelashes catch dust, dirt particles, or other things that could irritate our eyes, so our pubic hair catches things that could irritate the sensitive area between our outer lips. During childhood, we don't need the protection the pubic hair provides because this area is not as sensitive as it becomes during puberty.

Feelings About Pubic Hair

Some of the girls we talked to felt really excited about growing pubic hairs. Here's what one girl had to say:

> One day I was taking a bath and I noticed three little curly hairs growing down there. I started yelling for my mom to come and see. I felt real grown up.

Other girls weren't sure what was happening. As one girl explained.

> I saw these curly, black hairs and I didn't know what they were, so I got the tweezers and pulled them out. Pretty soon, they grew back, and then there were more and more of them. So I figured it must be okay.

Growing pubic hair can be pretty scary, especially if you don't know what's happening. A number of girls told us that they plucked their first pubic hairs. It's not really a very good idea to pluck your pubic hairs. For one thing, they'll just grow back. Also, plucking them could cause the skin to get irritated, sore, or infected (not to mention the fact that plucking them could be very painful).

Although many of the girls we talked to felt excited about beginning puberty, not all of them were. Some of the girls didn't like the fact that they were growing pubic hair and going through the other changes of puberty. One girl had this to say:

> I just wasn't ready. I remember when I first saw that my pubic hairs were growing. I thought, Oh, no, I don't want this to start happening to me yet. Then I got breasts and it was like I suddenly started having this grown-up body, but I still felt like a kid inside.

Another girl said that she was excited and proud about her body maturing, but at the same time, she was also uncertain:

> I was afraid I was going to have to be all grown up and wear high heels all the time instead of being a tomboy and climbing trees. But, really, it turned out that I did just the same things I always did.

All the girls we talked to, whether they felt good or bad (or a bit of both) about the changes happening in their bodies, agreed that it helps to have someone to talk to about your feelings. Reading this book with someone might be a good way of starting to talk about those things.

Underarm Hair

We also start to grow hair under our arms during puberty. Most girls don't start growing underarm hair until after they've started growing pubic hair or their breasts have started developing. Many don't grow underarm hair until after their first period. But for a few girls, underarm hair is the very first sign that puberty is beginning. Although this is unusual, it's not abnormal, and it doesn't mean there's anything wrong. The other changes, developing pubic hair and breasts and having your first period, will all happen eventually.

Other Body Hair

The hair on our arms and legs may get darker as we go through puberty, and we may have more of it than we did during childhood. Some girls notice that they begin to grow darker hairs on their upper lips as well.

Shaving

In some parts of the world, women with lots of under-arm and leg hair are considered more attractive or more womanly than women who don't have much hair on these parts of their bodies. In our country, the opposite seems to be true, at least in many people's minds. Here it seems that women who don't have hair on their underarms or legs are considered more attractive. The pretty, glamorous women we see in magazines, on TV, and in the movies have smooth, hairless legs and armpits. It's not that these women are somehow different from us and don't grow hair in these places. They are hairless because they shave their hair or they remove it by using chemical hair removers or by some other means.

Boys start growing hair under their arms and on their legs during puberty too. When boys start growing hair in these places, they generally feel very proud. It is a sign that they are turning from boys into men. On men, leg and underarm hair is considered attractive and manly. On women, it is often considered unattractive and unfeminine, which doesn't make much sense if you think about it.

You'll have to decide for yourself whether or not you want to remove the hair from your legs and underarms. It's not always easy to make this decision on your own because of pressure from the people around you, as in this girl's case.

> I wasn't going to shave my legs, but then my girlfriends started saying, "Oh, gross, look at all the hair on your legs. How come you don't shave it?" So I started doing it even though I didn't really want to.

Some girls said that they wanted to shave their legs, but their mothers said they couldn't. If your mom doesn't want you to shave and you want to, that's something you and she will have to work out between you. Your decision should be your own, though, without pressure one way or another from someone else. (We hope this last statement doesn't get us in trouble with too many moms.)

If you do decide to shave, there are a couple of things you should know before you start. If you remove the hair, it is apt to grow back darker and thicker. It also tends to grow back faster each time, so that after a few years, you may have to remove it every couple of days if you want to stay smooth.

If you do decide to remove the hair, you can shave it or use a chemical cream remover or a wax remover. If you shave, you can use an electric razor or the plain old-fashioned kind. Make sure the blades are smooth and free of nicks, or you'll cut yourself. A dull blade can pull at your skin and irritate, so make sure you've got a sharp one. It's pretty hard to cut yourself with an electric razor, but it's not at all hard to cut yourself with a regular one, so go easy. Use soap or shaving cream to cut down the pull or drag of the razor on your skin.

The chemical cream hair removers kill the hair at the root. You put the cream on and leave it there for a certain amount of time. When you wipe it off, the hair comes off too. Most cream removers can only be used on your legs. Don't use them on your armpits unless the instructions say it's safe to do so or you could get badly irritated or infected armpits. Never use a cream hair remover intended for your legs or armpits on your face. It could badly irritate the facial skin. Also be sure to follow the instructions and test the cream for an allergic reaction on a small area of skin before using it.

Another way of removing hair is to heat wax and spread it on the area where you want the hair removed. When the wax is cool, you pull it off and the hairs pull out with it. Drugstores sell these wax kits, but here again, make sure you follow instructions. Also, be sure the wax is intended for use on the area where you plan to use it.

If you develop dark hairs on your upper lip during puberty and want to remove them, don't use a razor or after awhile you'll have a stubble. There are chemical removers made for removing facial hair, but one woman we know told us that after a number of years the skin on her upper lip became slightly discolored from the chemical. Some women feel wax removers are better for removing hair from the upper lip. Other women prefer a more permanent method of removal known as electrolysis, in which an electric current is used to destroy the hair root. But even with electrolysis, the hair may grow back, and like the hair on your legs, it tends to grow back thicker and darker. So think twice about going through the hassle of removing it. If you really feel strongly about removing the hair from your upper lip, make an appointment with a doctor who specializes in skin problems (he or she is called a dermatologist) and ask the doctor to recommend the best method of hair removal for your skin type.

Perspiration

Another change you may notice as you go through puberty is that you begin to perspire (sweat) more. This is because your perspiration glands become more active during puberty. Your perspiration may take on an adult odor, too.

If you're eating good food and are healthy, your perspiration odor shouldn't be offensive. Taking a bath or shower every day should keep you smelling clean and fresh. If, however, the odor of your perspiration bothers you, there are any number of underarm deodorants that you can use. If you tend to perspire a great deal, you might want to use a deodorant that is also an anti-perspirant.

You also have sweat glands in your vulva and there are vaginal deodorants that you can use on your vulva. We don't recommend them though. They can be irritating to the sensitive skin in this area. Besides, unless you have an infection, a daily washing with soap and water should be all it takes to keep you smelling clean. If you have a strong-smelling discharge from your vagina and your vulva area smells bad, you may have an infection and should see a doctor rather than covering up the odor with a vaginal deodorant. (For more information on vaginal infections, see page 99.)

Pimples and Other Skin Problems

The oil glands in your skin also become more active and start producing more oil as you go through puberty. As the skin becomes more oily, most of us experience some skin problems. Pimples are the most common kind of skin problem. Almost everyone has at least a few as they are going through puberty. They usually show up on the face, shoulders, or the back. Pimples occur when the oil glands get clogged up with oil. They may get infected and become an angry, red color. Some boys and girls have very serious pimples and skin disturbances called acne. If you have acne, you may want to see a dermatologist.

It used to be thought that eating chocolate and greasy foods would cause you to have more pimples. Lately, doctors think that eating these foods doesn't have anything to do with pimples. About the best thing to do for pimples is to keep your face clean with soap and water.

Some people develop purplish marks on their skin, usually on the hips and buttocks, during puberty. These marks fade away as you grow into adulthood.

Pubic hair, underarm hair, skin changes, and perspiration are just a few of the differences your body will experience during puberty. In the next chapter we'll be talking about yet another change—the change in your breasts.

CHAPTER 4

Boobs, Boobies, Knockers, Melons, Jugs, Tits, and Titties: Your Breasts

Eskimos have over a hundred words for snow in their language because snow is such an important part of their lives. Judging from the number of words we have for breasts—the boys and girls in my class came up with dozens—breasts must be an important part of our lives.

I no longer remember exactly when I first noticed that my breasts were beginning to develop, but I sure remember the first time someone else noticed. I was baby-sitting for some friends of my parents who had nine-year-old twin girls. It was the first time I'd ever baby-sat for these girls. (It was also the last time. They dumped their pet guppies in the toilet, "so the guppies would have more room to swim around." While I was on my hands and knees fishing the guppies out of the toilet bowl, they were down in the kitchen putting their miniature turtle into the toaster, "to get it warmed up.")

The evening got off to a bad start. They were nice as pie while their mom and dad were there, but as soon as the door closed behind their parents, they jumped on me, pulling open my blouse: "Oh, you've got titties. Let's see, let's see," they demanded, "We can't wait till we get titties."

I managed to get the two of them off me and to button up my blouse, but I had never been so embarrassed in my life.

Regardless of whether you're as eager as those two twins or as mortified as I was, sooner or later your breasts will begin to develop.

The Breast during Childhood

When we are children, our breasts are flat, except for a small, raised portion in the center of each breast called the *nipple*. The nipple can range in color from a light pink to a brownish black and is surrounded by a

nipple (NIP-pull)

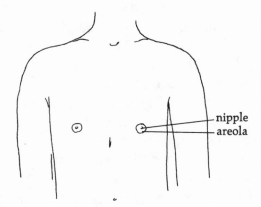

Illustration 10. The Breast. In the center of each breast is a small raised part called the "nipple," which is surrounded by a ring of skin called the "areola."

ring of flesh of about the same color that is called the *areola* (see Illustration 10).

Sometimes, when our breasts are touched or stroked or when we are feeling sexual, our nipples may stand out a little more, and the areola may pucker up and get bumpy. Otherwise, during childhood our breasts are flat and smooth, and only the nipple stands out. During puberty, the breasts begin to swell and to stand out more. The nipple and areola get larger and darker in color.

Inside the Breast

In order to understand why your breasts are swelling and beginning to stand out, you have to understand what is happening beneath the skin of your breast. Illustration 11 shows the inside of a grown woman's breast. Although you can only see three of them in this picture, a woman's breast is made up of fifteen to twenty-five separate parts, called *lobes*. The lobes are like the separate sections of an orange, all packed together inside the breast. They are surrounded by a cushion of fat. Inside each lobe is a sort of tree. The leaves of these trees are called *alveoli*. When a woman has a baby, milk is made inside these leaves. The milk travels from the leaves, through the branches and trunk of the tree, which are called milk ducts, to the nipple. When a mother breastfeeds, the baby sucks on the nipple and out comes the milk.

As you begin puberty, you start to develop milk ducts under your breasts and fat tissue forms around those ducts to protect them. These milk ducts and fat

areola (ah-REE-oh-la)
alveoli (al-VEE-oh-lie)

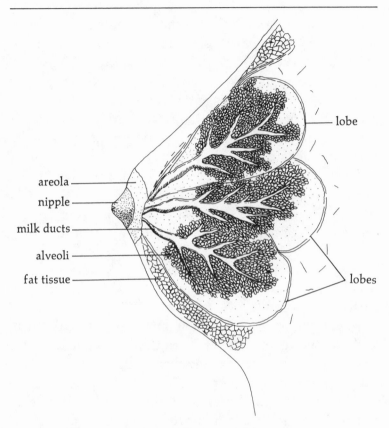

areola

nipple

milk ducts

alveoli

fat tissue

lobe

lobes

Illustration 11. Cross Section of an Adult Breast

tissue form a small mound under the nipple and areola called a *breast bud.* Your breasts are not yet ready to make milk and won't be able to do so until you have had a baby. But your body is beginning to get ready for the time when you may decide to have a baby, and this is what causes your breasts to swell and stand out.

Breast Development

No one can say for sure when a girl's breasts will start to develop. Sometimes it starts to happen when the girl is only eight and other times not until after she is sixteen or older. Most girls begin to develop breast buds between their ninth and fourteenth birthdays. But you may not be like most girls, so you may start earlier or later than this. Starting earlier or later than most girls does not mean there is anything wrong with you. It simply means that your body is growing at its own special rate.

Doctors have divided breast growth into five different stages that are pictured in Illustration 12. You may be in one of these stages or in between one stage and another. See if you can find the stage you're closest to.

Stage 1 shows how the breasts look during childhood. The breasts are flat, and the only part that is raised is the nipple.

Stage 2 is the breast-bud stage when the milk ducts and fat tissue form a small buttonlike mound under each nipple and areola, making them stick out. The nipple starts to get larger. This often happens just before the breast bud starts to form. The areola gets wider, and the nipple and areola get darker in color.

In Stage 3 the breasts get rounder and fuller and begin to stand out more. The nipple may continue to get larger and the areola wider. Both may get darker in color. The breasts are usually rather cone-shaped in this stage.

Stage 4 is a stage that many, but not all, girls go through. Girls who do go through it will notice that the areola and nipple form a separate little mound so that they stick out above the rest of the breast. Illustration 13 shows a closeup of the nipple and areola in Stage 3, Stage 4, and Stage 5 so you can see the difference more clearly.

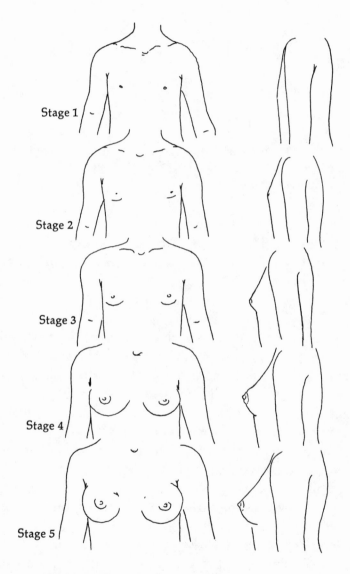

Illustration 12. The Five Stages of Breast Development

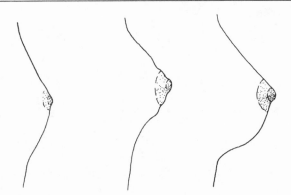

Illustration 13. Nipple in Stages 3, 4, 5. In stage 4, the nipple and areola form a separate mound so that they stick out from the general contour of the breast.

Stage 5 shows the grown-up, or adult, stage of breast development. The breasts are full and round. Some girls go directly from Stage 3 to Stage 5 without going through Stage 4.

Not only do breasts start developing at different ages, but they also develop at different rates. Some girls begin Stage 2, and within six months or a year they are already at Stage 5. Other girls take six or more years to go from Stage 2 to Stage 5. Most girls take about four and a half years to go from Stage 2 to Stage 5, but once again, you may not be like most girls, so you may take a longer or a shorter time.

Starting early or starting late doesn't have anything to do with how fast you will develop. Some girls start early and grow very fast, while other early starters develop slowly. Some girls who start late grow slowly, but other late starters develop very quickly.

Nor does starting early or starting late have anything to do with how big your breasts will be when you are fully grown. An early starter may wind up having either large or small breasts. The same is true for late starters—they may end up with large breasts or with small ones.

Breast Development and Your First Period

Most girls have their first menstrual period while they are in Stage 4 of breast development. However, a fair number will have their period while they are only in Stage 3, and some don't have their first period until after they've reached Stage 5. A few girls will have their first period while they are in Stage 2. If you have your first period while you are only in Stage 1 (before your breasts have begun to develop), you should see a doctor. Having your period before your breasts have begun to develop doesn't necessarily mean that something's wrong, but it *may* mean that you have a problem that needs a doctor's attention.

Feelings About Developing Breasts

The mothers and daughters we talked to all had different kinds of feelings about their breasts. Some girls were really excited when their breasts started developing, like this girl who told us:

> I was so happy when my breasts started growing. First my nipples got bigger. Then my breasts started sticking out. I was so proud. I felt real grown up. I was always showing them off to my mom and my little sister.

Although many girls feel excited, they also worry about one thing or another. One girl said:

> I was really freaked out. I had these little flat bumps under my nipples, and they hurt all the time, especially if they got hit or something. They were so sore. I thought maybe something was wrong.

One or both of your breasts *may* feel tender, sore, or downright painful at times. This is perfectly normal, and it doesn't mean that anything is wrong. Although it may be a bit uncomfortable, this soreness isn't anything to worry about. It's just part of growing up.

One question that regularly comes out of my class question box is "Could a girl's breasts burst?" or, as one girl wrote, "Could a girl's boobs pop like a balloon?" Each time I get one of these questions, I always answer, "No, that can't happen," but secretly I've always wondered where in the world anyone could have gotten an idea like that. Then one day, one of the girls came up after class and explained:

> Grown-ups are always saying things like, "Oh, you're really popping out," or "You're sure bursting out all over," and sometimes my breasts feel sore, like they really are about to burst, so I wondered.

This girl made me realize how confusing the things adults say can sound to kids sometimes. If you've worried about this same thing, you can stop worrying. I can asure you that even though it may feel that way at times, your breasts won't pop or burst.

Other girls we talked to told us that they worried because both their breasts didn't develop at the same rate. One girl said:

> One of my breasts was starting to grow, and the other one was still completely flat. I was afraid that the other one would never grow, and I was only going to have one breast instead of two.

Another girl explained:

> Both of mine started growing at the same time, but one of mine was a lot bigger than the other one, and I was worried that I was going to grow up all lopsided.

It often happens that one breast develops before the other or that one seems to be growing at a much faster rate than the other. Even though one may start growing first, the other will eventually grow too. By the time a girl is fully developed, both breasts are pretty much the same size. Many grown women do notice that one breast is slightly larger than the other, but this difference in size is generally too small to be noticed by anyone other than the woman herself.

Some girls notice that tiny hairs begin to develop around the areola. One of the girls that this happened to told us:

> I started growing these little hairs around my nipple, and none of my friends did. I thought I was weird, so I plucked them out with tweezers, but they just grew back.

Although most women don't grow hairs like this, many do. It's quite normal. Plucking these hairs doesn't usually get rid of them, for most of the time they just grow back. In fact, plucking them out could cause problems, for it might start an infection that could make your breast sore, red, and painful.

"One of my nipples didn't stick out and the other did," yet another girl told us. "It sort of puckered in, and I wondered why."

This girl had what is known as an inverted nipple. One or both nipples in some girls and women sink into the areola instead of sticking out. As a girl grows older, the inverted nipple may start to stick out. Lots of women have inverted nipples. They don't cause any problems. You may have heard that women with inverted nipples can't breastfeed their babies. This is simply not true. The only time that inverted nipples might be a problem is if a nipple that wasn't inverted suddenly becomes inverted, or vice versa. This doesn't necessarily mean that anything is wrong, but it is something to check out with your doctor.

Some girls we talked to worried because they noticed a little fluid coming from their nipples once in awhile. This is normal. It is your body's way of keeping your ducts open. The fluid may be whitish or clear or slightly yellow or green. If there is a lot of it or if it is dark brown or has pus in it, see your doctor, for it may be a sign of an infection. (We'll talk more about inverted nipples and fluids coming out of the nipples later on when we talk about breast self-exam.)

As we said earlier, many of the girls we talked to felt excited and proud about developing breasts, but many also felt uncomfortable or embarrassed. A twenty-two-year-old told us:

> I was only in fourth grade when I started developing, and no one else was. I used to wrap one of those bandages, the kind you put on a sprained ankle, around my chest to make me flat. I kept my coat on as much as I could and wore baggy clothes all the time. Now that I'm older, I can laugh about it, but back then it wasn't funny at all.

Many of the girls and women whose breasts started developing earlier than most talked about feeling embarrassed. Girls whose breasts began to develop late often had embarrassed feelings too. One woman, now in her thirties, told us:

> I didn't start to develop until after my sixteenth birthday. Everyone, and I mean *everyone*, had breasts but me. They were all in their bras, and there I was in my undershirt. I flunked gym in high school because I wouldn't take a shower. I was too embarrassed about my flat chest. Finally, my mom bought me a padded bra. My breasts did eventually start to develop, but I really felt bad about myself for a lot of years before they did.

Another woman told us:

> I didn't start developing until I was seventeen. I thought
> there was something horribly wrong, like maybe I was
> really a man instead of a woman. Oh, and the teasing I
> had to endure! The boys used to call me "ironing board"
> because my chest was so flat.

Even girls who were neither early nor late starters
feel embarrassed. As one girl put it:

> I started to develop when I was eleven, just about the
> same time as everyone else. I was glad that I was getting
> tits, but I was embarrassed, especially at school.

Our parents, our brothers and sisters, our friends,
people at school may tease us about developing breasts,
and this may make us feel embarrassed at times. Even
strangers, people on the street, may make comments on
our changing bodies. Boys or men may whistle or make
sexual remarks. Sometimes this attention is flattering.
As one girl explained:

> If I'm walking down the street and some guy says, "Hey,
> there!" or whistles or something, I feel pretty good, like
> he's saying, "Oh, you look good," especially if I'm with
> a girlfriend or a bunch of girls.

But a lot of girls and women don't like this kind of
attention:

> I hate when boys stare at my breasts or whistle or yell
> stuff at me. It makes me feel like a piece of meat, and
> it makes me feel self-conscious and dumb. I mean, what
> can you do? Yell back at them? How would they like it
> if girls went down the street and stared at their crotches
> and yelled stuff like, "Hey, that's a really big penis you
> got there!" Boys do that. They say stuff like, "Hey,
> that's a great set of jugs!" I don't like it.

Often there isn't much you can do about this unwanted attention, beyond simply ignoring it. But it may be helpful to talk about these experiences with other girls so you can help each other deal with such situations.

Bras

We get a lot of questions about when a girl should start wearing a bra or if she even needs to wear one at all. Thre are no clear-cut answers to this; it's something you have to decide for yourself. If you have small breasts or very firm ones, you may not need a bra. But if you have large breasts, you may decide to wear a bra for reasons of comfort. Also, some girls wear bras because when you get older your breasts may begin to droop if they haven't been well supported. One girl in our classes had something interesting to say about this:

> So what if your breasts droop? I mean, who says that breasts that don't droop are better than breasts that do? I don't care. I don't wear a bra and I'm not going to. I hate the way they feel, like I'm in a harness or something.

Some girls said they wear bras because they feel more comfortable having some support, so their breasts don't joggle around when they run or dance or play sports. Others told us that they wear bras because they feel self-conscious without them. The best rule to follow is to do whatever feels best for you.

Bras come in different sizes. There are "training bras" for girls whose breasts are just beginning to develop. They are usually made of a stretchy material so that they will fit even if your breasts have hardly developed at all. Regular bras, those that aren't training bras, come in various cup sizes (the cup is the part of the bra that fits over the breast). The smallest cup size is a triple A (AAA) or a double A (AA). Then comes an A, then a B size cup, a C, a D, an E and sometimes a very large double E. Bras also come marked in different inches ranging from about twenty-eight inches to forty-four inches or more. You can tell how many inches you need by measuring around your body just under your breasts, as you see in Illustration 14. If you measure thirty inches, you'll need a thirty-inch bra. If your breasts are just beginning to develop, you'll probably need a triple or double A, so you'd ask for a thirty-inch triple A or a thirty-inch double A. You can buy bras in most department stores, and the salesperson will measure you and help you select the proper size and style.

You may have heard about padded bras and "falsies." Padded bras are bras that have a pad of cotton or foam rubber on the inside of the cup. When you put on a padded bra it appears that your breasts are larger than they really are. "Falsies" are breast-shaped inserts

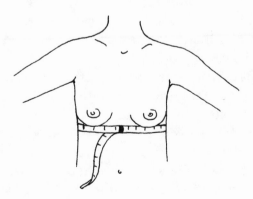

Illustration 14. Measuring for a Bra. To determine your bra size, measure yourself with a tape measure, as shown here.

that are worn inside the cup of a bra—again, to make it seem as if your breasts are larger than they actually are.

Breast Size

When I was a girl, we used to do an exercise in gym class where we'd hold our arms at shoulder level, elbows bent, and jerk our elbows back to a one-two, one-two count. While we did this exercise, we chanted:

> *We must, we must,*
> *We must increase our busts.*
> *It's better, it's better,*
> *It's better for the sweater.*
> *We may, we may,*
> *We may get big someday.*

I hope girls no longer have to do this in gym class, not that there's anything wrong with the exercise. It's a good exercise for toning and firming the muscles of the chest wall. (It won't, however, make your breasts larger. Your breasts are composed of glands and fat tissue and no amount of exercise will enlarge them. If you do this exercise a lot, the chest muscles underneath the breast will get thicker and this will make your breasts stand out more.)

No, there's nothing wrong with the exercise itself, it's the chant that went along with it—all that business about "we must increase our busts" and the emphasis on having big breasts, as if big breasts were somehow better than small ones. Breasts feel the same and can give us the same pleasurable feelings when they are stroked or touched regardless of their size. Small breasts do just as good a job of making breast milk as large ones. Still with all the big-busted, glamorous women in advertisements, films, and TV shows, it's easy to get the idea that big breasts are more womanly or more sexy than small ones. But despite all the advertising, there are a great many people who find small breasts equally, if not more, attractive than large ones. And anyone who decides whether he or she likes you or not because of the size of your breasts probably isn't a person worth knowing anyhow.

Still, we do live in a country that has a hang-up about breasts. Some women with small breasts who feel self-conscious may have a difficult time, which is why there are padded bras and falsies and operations to enlarge breasts. If padded bras or falsies sound like the right choice for you, you can find them in the bra section of any department store and the salesclerk will help fit you. Breast size can be a problem for large-breasted women too. Some women have such large breasts that it affects their posture and causes back pains. Having tremendously big breasts can be embarrassing too. If you have this problem, you should know that there are also operations to reduce breasts to a more comfortable size. Operations to reduce or enlarge breasts can't be done, however, until you are fully grown because your breasts are still developing and the operation could interfere with normal development.

Regardless of whether your breasts are large or small or medium-size, it's important that you learn how to practice breast self-exam.

Breast Self-Exam

Breast self-exam, called BSE for short, means examining your breasts to see if there are any lumps or other irregularities that might be signs of breast cancer.

Not all breast lumps are signs of cancer. In fact, the

vast majority of lumps that women find in their breasts are *not* cancerous. But since cancer can appear as a small lump in the breast, it is important to examine your breasts and have a doctor check any lumps you do find to rule out the possibility of breast cancer.

One out of every fourteen women in the country gets breast cancer. In some cases, breast cancer can be cured by removing the lump. Other times, it is necessary to remove the whole breast. Sometimes, breast cancer can't be cured and the woman dies. If a woman discovers her breast cancer while the lump is small, she has a much better chance of being cured. That's why breast self-exam is so important. If a woman feels her breasts regularly, once a month, she has a better chance of being able to find the lump right away, before the cancer is so serious that it can't be cured.

Actually, breast exam is not real important for teen-agers because teen-agers don't, as a rule, get breast cancer. (There have been a few young women who've had breast cancer, but it's very rare.) Many doctors tell women to start examining their breasts after they've reached their twenty-fifth birthdays, since breast cancer is rare before the age of twenty-five.

We suggest that young women start examining their breasts as soon as they have had their first menstrual periods. We think this is a good idea for two reasons. First of all, it gets you started, while you're young, on what should become a lifelong habit. But perhaps more importantly, if you're examining your breasts regularly, it might get your mom, your older sisters, or other women you may live with to do it too. Far too many women neglect this live-saving measure. Maybe your doing it will set an example for them. Why don't you and your mom or another adult woman try practicing breast exam, which is described below, together?

Breast exam should be done about once a month. The best time is right after your menstrual period is over. Some women's breasts tend to be a little lumpy before or during their menstrual periods because the ducts and tissues of the breast swell a bit. If you are one of these women, you will find that your breasts are less lumpy just after your period, so it will be easier to do the exam at that time.

Breast exam should be done when you are relaxed and are not feeling rushed. The exam consists of two parts: 1) looking at your breasts, and 2) feeling them.

PART ONE: LOOKING (ILLUSTRATION 15)

To begin, stand in front of a well-lighted mirror with your arms down at your sides and take a good look at your breasts from the front and from each side. Look to see if there are any depressions, bulges, moles, dimples, dark or red areas, swellings, sores, or areas of skin with a rough or orange peel-like texture. Check the nipple and areola as well as the skin of the breast. If you have any of these problems, keep an eye on them and if they're not gone in a couple of weeks, see a doctor. At your age, these problems aren't likely to be signs of cancer, but you may have a noncancerous problem in your breast that needs attention.

Next, put your hands on your hips and press inward and down so that the muscles of your upper chest tighten. Check to see if the muscles contract about the same amount or if any bulging or dimpling shows up on your breasts when you've got your muscles tight like this. Sometimes, a lump that isn't noticeable in the first position will become obvious only when you tighten. While your hands are still on your hips, rotate to each side, looking for the same things.

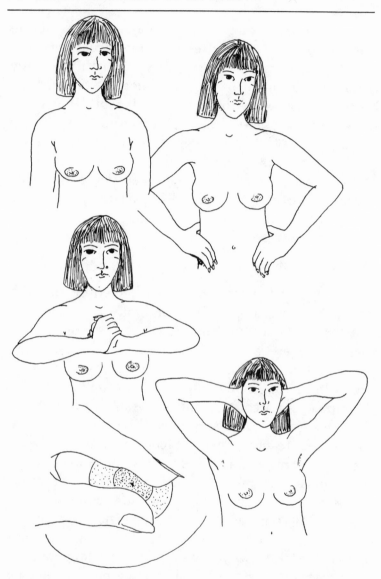

Illustration 15. Breast Self-Exam, Part One: Looking. Stand in front of a mirror and inspect your breasts in each of the four positions shown here. Finally, squeeze each nipple for signs of discharge.

Now put your arms in front of your chest at about heart level, press your palms together, and check for uneven muscle contraction, bulges, or dimpling. Check each side of your breasts. If your breasts are large or hang down, you may have to lift each breast to check the underside.

Next raise your arms, bend your elbows, and place your hands behind your head. Once again, check from the front and from both sides for any signs of dimpling or bulging that might indicate a lump or thickening inside the breast.

To finish the first part of the exam, gently squeeze each nipple to see if you can get any fluid to come out. Fluid from the nipple is not necessarily a sign that something is wrong. But if there is a lot of it or if it is dark in color or full of pus, see a doctor.

PART TWO: FEELING (ILLUSTRATION 16)

This part is done lying down because when you lie down your breasts spread out and it will be easier to feel for lumps. Lotion or oil will make your fingers more sensitive.

To begin, bend one arm and place your hand behind your head. Use the fatty pads of your fingers rather than your fingertips, and starting on the outside of your breast, using a circular motion, carefully feel each breast. Press all the way down to the chest wall. Also feel the upper part of your chest and under your armpit. Repeat the process on the other side.

What you are looking, or rather, feeling for, is any lump or thickening in the breast, the chest, or under the armpits. This sounds pretty simple, but it can be tricky. For one thing, it's kind of like feeling for a

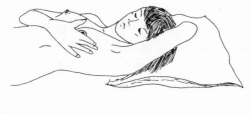

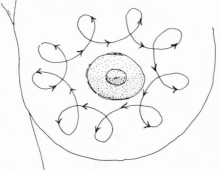

Illustration 16. Breast Self-Exam, Part Two: Feeling. Lie down with one hand behind your head. With your other hand, start on the outside of your breast and, using a circular motion, feel the entire breast. Repeat on the opposite breast.

marble in a bag filled with jello. Every time you press near it, the lump moves away. You may have to use two hands now and then to support your breast in order to get a good feel. It's also hard because most women have rather bumpy or even lumpy breasts. It's easy to mistake the ducts, the ribs, the breastbone, or the underlying muscles for lumps. Once you have been doing it for a while, though, you'll be able to tell the difference between the normal lumps and bumps and any abnormal ones.

If you find any lumps, thickening, red spots, bulges, or unusual fluid from your nipples, or if a nipple suddenly becomes inverted (or if an inverted nipple suddenly begins to stick out), *don't panic.* Remember, breast cancer in young women is very, very rare. But there are other, noncancerous conditions that can affect young girls' breasts. So, if your symptoms last more than two weeks, get them checked out.

CHAPTER 5

Changes in the Vulva

The genital organs on the outside of your body, which are sometimes referred to as the vulva, also change as you go through puberty. The various parts of the vulva are easy to see if you hold a mirror between your legs as the girl in Illustration 17 is doing. The other drawings in Illustration 17 show how the vulva looks in a young girl, in a young woman going through puberty, and in a grown woman.

The easiest way to learn about these organs and how they change during puberty is to use a mirror and compare your own body to these drawings. You probably won't look exactly like any of these drawings because each person's body is a little bit different. But if you looked at a drawing of a person's face with eyes, a nose, a mouth, and so on, you could easily find the eyes, nose, or mouth on your own face, even if the drawing didn't look *exactly* like your own face. In the

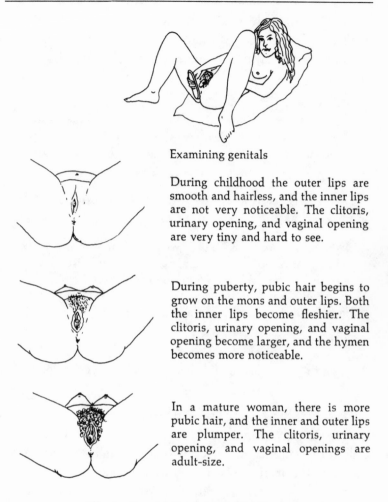

Examining genitals

During childhood the outer lips are smooth and hairless, and the inner lips are not very noticeable. The clitoris, urinary opening, and vaginal opening are very tiny and hard to see.

During puberty, pubic hair begins to grow on the mons and outer lips. Both the inner lips become fleshier. The clitoris, urinary opening, and vaginal opening become larger, and the hymen becomes more noticeable.

In a mature woman, there is more pubic hair, and the inner and outer lips are plumper. The clitoris, urinary opening, and vaginal openings are adult-size.

Illustration 17. Examining the Genitals

same way, you can look at a drawing of a vulva and find the various parts on your own vulva. Of course, we're a lot more used to looking at faces than vulvas, but with a little practice, you can learn to see the features of your vulva as plainly as you can see the nose on your face.

Some people think that using a mirror to look at this area of their bodies, touching the various parts, and learning their names is a dandy idea. As one girl in our class said:

> Oh, I've looked at myself there lots of times. My mom got a mirror and showed me how to look at myself and how she looked so I'd know what I'll look like when I grow up. She taught me the names of everything and all that stuff.

Other girls don't feel as comfortable about touching or looking at their genitals. One girl in our class said:

> I thought it sounded kind of weird, taking a mirror and looking at myself down there, but I was kind of curious, so I locked my bedroom door and took a good look. I'm glad I did, 'cause it made me feel like I know more about myself, like it wasn't such a big mystery.

Still another girl said:

> Ugh, that's disgusting. I'd never do that. It's yucky down there.

This girl had been taught that her genitals were dirty and ugly and that it was shameful or wrong to look at or touch them. Even if no one has never actually said to you that there is something wrong or dirty about your genitals, you may still feel uncertain about exploring them. People don't talk about genital organs very much, and as we all know, if something is too terrible to talk about, then it's probably really terrible!

But there is nothing terrible or wrong about this area of your body. People feel uncomfortable because it is a sexual part of the body, and people often feel uncomfortable about anything that has to do with sex. Some people get the idea that this part of the body is dirty because the openings through which urine and feces leave our bodies are located here. Actually, this area of our bodies isn't any dirtier than, say, the inside of our mouths. (In fact, our mouths have more germs than this area of our bodies.)

In the following pages, we'll take you on a guided tour of the vulva and explain how your genitals change during puberty. If you don't feel comfortable about touching or looking at your genitals, that's fine. Just read these pages and look at the pictures. We wouldn't want you to do anything you don't feel okay doing. If you'd like to, though, we think you'll find it helpful to keep a mirror handy so you can look at yourself as you read about these parts of your body. You may want to do this all by yourself, with a friend, or with your mom. Do whatever feels most comfortable for you.

The Mons

We'll start our tour at the top of the vulva, at the mons. As you may remember, the mons is a pad of fat tissue that covers the pubic bone. It is here, on the mons, that pubic hair begins to grow during puberty, and in grown women the mons is covered with curly pubic hair.

In addition to sprouting hair, the mons also gets fleshier during puberty so that it sticks out more. This is because the fat pad over the pubic bone is getting thicker.

The Outer Lips

As you move down along the mons, you will see that it divides into two separate flaps, or folds, of skin. As we told you earlier, these are the outer lips, or the labia majora. *Labia* is a Latin word meaning lips and *majora* means major, so they are sometimes called the "major lips."

In a young girl, the outer lips may be hairless, or they may have a few light-colored hairs. During puberty, pubic hair begins to grow on the outer lips.

In young girls, the lips are often separated. There may be space between them, so they may not actually touch each other. During puberty, the lips get fleshier and they often begin to touch. In grown women, the lips generally touch, but some women find that after they've had a baby, the lips are slightly separated again. In very old women, the lips get thinner, less fleshy, and may become separated again.

The lips are usually smooth in a young girl, but during puberty, they may get sort of wrinkly. In grown women, they tend to be wrinkly. Many women find that when they are old and gray, the lips get smooth again.

The outer lips help protect the area underneath. The underside of the lips are hairless, both in young girls and in grown women. In girls, the underside of the lips are smooth, but as you go through puberty, you may notice small, slightly raised bumps dotting the skin on the underside of the lips. These are oil glands. They make a small amount of oil that keeps the area moist so that it doesn't get irritated. Once you start puberty, you may notice a slight feeling of wetness in this area because of this oil. You may also notice a change in the way this area of your body smells. Again, this is because of the oil made by these glands.

During childhood, this area may be light pink to red to brownish-black in color, depending on your skin tone. The color is apt to change during puberty, getting either lighter or darker.

The Inner Lips

If you separate the outer lips, you will see two ridges, or folds, of skin called the *labia minora*, the minor lips, or the little lips. During childhood, the inner lips may not be very noticeable, but during puberty, they grow and become more noticeable. Like the outer lips, they protect the area between them, and they too tend to change color and get more wrinkly during puberty.

As you can see in Illustration 18, the labia look different in different women. In most women, the inner lips are smaller than the outer lips, but in some women, the inner lips protrude beyond the outer lips. The inner lips are usually about the same size, but some women notice that one is larger than the other.

The inner lips are hairless in both girls and grown women. They tend to be more moist as we grow older because they too have oil glands that begin producing more oil during puberty.

The Clitoris

If you follow the inner lips up toward the mons, you will see that they join together at the top. In the area where the inner lips join together lies the tip of the clitoris, in slang terms, the "clit." In grown women, the clitoris is about the size of the eraser on the end of a pencil. The way in which the inner lips join together is not the same in all women. In some women, the inner lips come together forming a sort of hood that covers the clitoris. In other women, the clitoris sticks all or part

minora (mi-NOR-ah)

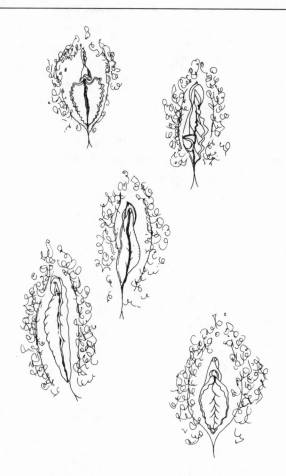

Illustration 18. The Labia. The inner lips look different in different women.

of the way out from the folds of the hood formed by the inner lips. When we are feeling sexual, the clitoris tends to swell and get a little large for a while. It also grows permanently larger during puberty.

You may have to pull back the hood formed by the inner lips in order to see the clitoris; even then you can only see the tip of the clitoris. The rest of the clitoris lies buried under the skin. If you press down on the skin above the clitoris, you may be able to feel a rubbery cord under the skin. This is the shaft of the clitoris.

Masturbation

The clitoris and its shaft—in fact, this whole area of your body—is very sensitive. When you touch it, you may get an excited, tingly kind of feeling. Touching, rubbing, stroking, or squeezing this area of your body so that you will have these feelings is called *masturbating* or *masturbation*. There are also lots of slang words for masturbation, such as "jerking off," "playing with yourself," or "jacking off."

Sometimes when people masturbate, they get so excited that they have a shivery feeling that is called an *orgasm*. Having an orgasm is also called "coming" or "climaxing." It's hard to explain exactly what an orgasm feels like, and orgasms probably feel different to different people, but most people agree that it is a good feeling.

Not everyone masturbates, but many if not most of us do at some time or other in our lives. Some women start masturbating when they are children and continue to do so all their lives. Some start during puberty; others don't start until they are grown women. Still others never masturbate. It's normal if you do it and normal if you don't.

You may have heard all sorts of strange things about masturbation. People used to think that masturbation would make you insane or make you go blind or turn you into a moron. Obviously, these things aren't true

masturbating (MASS-tur-bait-ing)
masturbation (MASS-tur-bay-shun)
orgasm (or-GAZ-um)
climaxing (KLY-max-ing)

or there would be an awful lot of insane, blind morons around. You may have heard that masturbation would cause you to grow hair on the palms of your hands, pimples on your face, warts on your fingers, or other terrible things. Again, none of this is true. You may have heard that masturbation will make you enjoy sex with another person less: also not true. Actually, masturbating is a way of rehearsing for your adult sex life. By learning how to give yourself pleasure sexually, you are taking the first step in learning how to have sexual pleasure with someone else.

One question that frequently comes up in our classes is whether or not masturbating "too much" can hurt you in some way. The answer is no. Nothing bad will happen to your body regardless of how much you masturbate; masturbation is not harmful in any way. About the only thing that can happen is that your genitals might get a little sore if you are masturbating and rubbing them a whole lot. Some people masturbate every day. Some masturbate many times in one day. Others only rarely masturbate, and still others never do. Remember, it's normal if you do it and normal if you don't.

Some people like to imagine things that make them feel more excited when they are masturbating. Imagining or pretending that something is happening is called daydreaming or fantasizing. We daydream and fantasize about all sorts of things. When our daydreams are about sexual things, we call them sexual fantasies. Almost everyone has sexual fantasies. Fantasies are a rich and varied way of experimenting with your sexual self. They are perfectly okay, so relax and enjoy them. But let's leave the subjects of masturbation and sexual fantasies and get back to the guided tour of your body.

The Urinary Opening

If you move down your clitoris in a straight line, you will come to the urinary opening. *Urinary* comes from the word *urine*. Urine is made inside our bodies. The food we eat and drink is broken down inside of us so that our bodies can use it. Not everything we eat and drink can be used by our bodies. After everything is broken down and used, some of the leftovers are in the form of the clear, yellowish, waterlike liquid called urine. The urine collects in an organ inside our bodies called the *bladder*. The bladder is like a balloon or bag. It has a small tube at the bottom, which leads to the outside of our bodies. The urinary opening is the outside end of this tube. When our bladder is full, we press down, the tube opens up, and the urine from the bladder runs down the tube and out through the urinary opening.

It may be difficult for you to see exactly where the urinary opening is. If you start at the clitoris and move downward in a straight line, the first dimpled area you come to is the urinary opening. It may look like an upside down V. During puberty, the urinary opening becomes more noticeable than it is during childhood.

If you don't stay on a straight line down from the clitoris, you may mistake the opening to one of the two tiny glands also located in this area for the urinary opening. The opening to these glands are two little slits on either side of the urinary opening. Like the oil glands on the inner and outer lips, these glands make a small amount of oil that keeps this area moist. Some women have such tiny openings to these glands that they can't be seen; others have larger ones that can be mistaken for the urinary opening.

The Vaginal Opening

Now that you know where the urinary opening is, you'll be able to find the vaginal opening. As we explained earlier, the vagina is up inside your body, so you won't be able to see the vagina itself, but you will be able to find the opening to the vagina. If you move down from the urinary opening—again, in a straight line—you'll come to the vaginal opening.

Pictures of the vaginal opening are sometimes confusing since they make it look as if the vaginal opening is a dark, gaping hole. It's not. The vagina itself is like a pouch. In young girls, it's not very big. During puberty, it starts to grow, but even in adult women, it's about four or five inches long. But the vagina is like a balloon, and it can expand to many times its size. It has to be able to expand like this so a man's penis can fit in there during sexual intercourse. Also, when a woman has a baby, the baby travels through the vagina on its way out of the mother's body.

Most of the time, though, the sides of the vagina touch each other. If you were to look into the opening of a collapsed balloon, you wouldn't see an empty space. You'd see the collapsed sides of the balloon all folded up and touching each other. The same is true of the vagina: When you look into the vaginal opening, you don't see a hole, you see the fleshy walls of the vagina up against each other.

The Hymen

The vaginal opening may be partly covered by a thin piece of skin just inside the opening called the *hymen.*

hymen (HI-men)

Other names for the hymen are "cherry" or "maiden-head." The hymen looks different in different women. It may just be a thin fringe of skin around the edges of the vaginal opening. It may stretch across the opening with one or more holes in it. Illustration 19 shows just a few of the ways the hymen may look.

In young girls, the hymen may not be very noticeable. During puberty, it usually gets thicker and more rigid and more noticeable. Not everyone has a hymen. Some women are born without one. Other women's hymens are so torn and stretched that it's hard to see them.

As strange as it seems, some people used to think that this tiny little piece of skin was *very, very* important. People thought that all women had the kind of hymens that only have a few holes and that stretch across the vaginal opening. They thought that the only way a hymen could be stretched or torn was if a man put his penis inside a woman's vagina while they were having sex. Today we know this isn't true. Not all

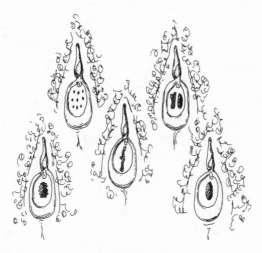

Illustration 19. The Hymen. The hymen may have one or two large openings or several small ones.

women have hymens and, of those who do, not all have the kind that stretch across the vaginal opening. Some have such small, thin ones that they are hardly noticeable. Also, hymens can get stretched or torn in a number of ways. Horseback riding, doing a split, falling off a bike—any stretching movement can tear the hymen. So not having a hymen or having one that has been stretched or torn doesn't have anything to do with whether or not a woman has had sex with a man. In fact, some women have sex with men without their hymens stretching or tearing at all.

But in the old days, people thought that if a woman didn't have an untorn, unstretched hymen covering her vaginal opening, this meant that she had already had sex with a man and was not a virgin (a virgin is a woman who has never had sex). People also thought that it was important that a woman be a virgin when she married. Many people still feel this way, but back then a woman who was not a virgin when she got married could get into a lot of trouble. In some countries, a woman could even be put to death if she wasn't a virgin when she married. In other countries, young women were examined before marriage to see if they had a hymen. If they didn't, the marriage could be called off. In still other countries, a bride was supposed to hang her bedsheets out the window the morning after her wedding night. Since her wedding night was the first time she was supposed to have sex, and since people thought the hymen would break and bleed only in sexual intercourse, the bride's bedsheets were supposed to have blood on them as proof to everyone that she had been a virgin before her wedding night.

You can imagine the problems all this fuss about the hymen made for those women who were born without hymens, for those whose hymens had been stretched or torn during childhood, or for those whose hymens simply weren't very noticeable. Some were killed and others never married or lived their lives in disgrace. Not only that, but some women's hymens don't bleed very much when they are stretched or torn. So, even those brides who were lucky enough to have hymens of the approved kind might not have had any blood on their wedding sheets. History is full of stories of clever brides who took a bit of animal's blood and poured it on the sheets to fool everyone. Still, it seems an awful lot of fuss about what is only a thin piece of skin.

People have, for the most part, changed their attitudes about the hymen. But, in some parts of the world, these ideas still persist, and you may have heard some of these stories. If so, just ignore them. Your hymen has nothing to do with whether or not you have had sex and neither a doctor nor anyone else can tell by looking at your body whether or not you've had sex.

When your hymen is stretched or torn—whether it's during sex or while you're doing gymnastics or riding a horse or whatever—it may bleed a little, a whole lot, or not at all. It may hurt a little, a whole lot, or not at all. If it does hurt a lot or bleed a whole lot, you should, of course, see your doctor. But only rarely does a hymen bleed or hurt so badly that a doctor's care is needed. Most women never notice any blood or feel anything when their hymens are stretched or torn.

The Anus

Although it is not really a sex organ, there is another opening in this area of the body called the *anus*. You have probably heard some of the slang terms like "asshole," "butthole," or "poophole" that are also used to refer to this opening.

If you continue moving down from the vaginal opening, you'll come to the anus. It is the outside opening to the bowels, which are long, hollow tubes that are coiled up inside of the body. The bowels are also called the *small intestines*.

Remember when we talked about how the food we take into our bodies is broken down and how urine is part of what is left over? Well, in addition to the watery urine, there are also more solid leftovers, which are called *feces*. People sometimes use slang words like "shit" or "poop" to refer to feces. The feces travel through the bowels and when we go to the bathroom and have a bowel movement, the feces come out through the anus.

The skin around the anus, just like the skin of the labia, may change color during puberty, getting a little darker. Pubic hair may also start to grow around the anus during puberty.

This completes the tour of the sex organs on the outside of your body. In the next chapter we will look at the inside of your body and still more changes that take place during puberty.

intestines (in-TES-tins)

CHAPTER 6

Changes in the Reproductive Organs

The changes occurring outside your body during puberty—the breast buds, the pubic hair, the changes in your vulva—happen because other, even more dramatic changes are taking place on the inside. In order to understand puberty and menstruation, you have to have some idea of what's going on inside you.

The Reproductive Organs

Just as we have sex organs on the outside of our bodies, so we have sex organs on the inside. The sex organs inside of our bodies are called reproductive organs because they are involved in the process of reproducing, that is, in having babies. Illustration 20 shows a side view of the reproductive organs—the vagina, uterus, tubes, and ovaries—in a young girl and in a grown woman. As you can see from these drawings, our re-cross section of reproductive organs in young girl

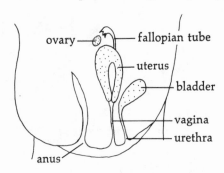

ovary — fallopian tube

uterus

bladder

vagina

urethra

anus

cross section of reproductive organs in older woman

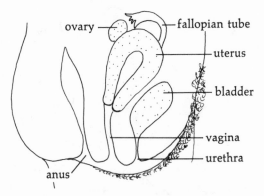

ovary — fallopian tube

uterus

bladder

vagina

urethra

anus

Illustration 20. Cross Section of Reproductive Organs. Our reproductive organs change as we get older. They grow larger and also change positions as they grow. Note that the uterus is almost vertical in a young girl, but is tilted forward in a woman.

productive organs also change as we get older. In this chapter we'll be talking about the changes that take place in these organs during puberty.

The Vagina

In the last chapter, you learned where the opening to your vagina is located. As we explained, the vagina itself is inside the body. The vagina is rather like a pouch

tucked up inside us, which is very elastic or stretchy so that a man's penis can fit inside it during sexual intercourse. It is so stretchable that it can expand to allow a baby to pass from the uterus and through the vagina during childbirth. Most of the time, though, the vagina is like a collapsed balloon without any air in it, and the inside walls of the vagina are all folded up and touching each other.

The vagina, like the other organs in our bodies, grows during childhood. And, like other parts of our bodies, it undergoes a growth spurt during puberty, so that it suddenly starts becoming longer until it reaches its adult length of four to five inches.

If you put your finger up inside your vagina, you'll be able to feel the soft, squishy vaginal walls all folded up against each other.

The idea of putting your finger up inside your vagina might seem a little weird. Many girls, and women too, are afraid that they might hurt themselves or injure themselves in some way by doing this. But there's nothing mysterious or breakable in there. You could no more injure yourself by putting a finger inside your vagina than you could by putting a finger inside your mouth. However, your vaginal opening and hymen may be rather small and tight, so it's possible that it might feel a bit uncomfortable to you, especially if you are feeling a bit nervous about exploring yourself in this way. There's a simple rule to follow here: If it hurts too much, don't do it. Using some K-Y Jelly or petroleum jelly might help make it easier, but don't use body lotions or other skin creams that have perfumes and chemicals added, as they could be irritating. If the opening to your vagina is so tight and small that it's hard to get your finger in there, you might want to slowly stretch the opening over a period of a few weeks

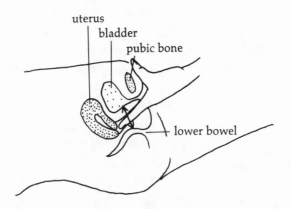

Illustration 21. The Vagina. If you press up toward the mons, you may feel the pubic bone and the urethra, the tube through which urine travels from the bladder. If you press down, you may feel lumps of feces in the lower bowel.

or months. Running your finger around the opening from time to time (while you're taking a hot bath is a good time) will help stretch it.

If you press upward, just inside the vaginal opening you'll feel a bone covered by a soft bulge of tissue. It may feel rather sensitive, for underneath this bulge lies the urethra, the tube that runs from the bottom of the bladder to the outside of your body. Pressing upward in this manner may give you the feeling that you have to urinate because the bladder lies quite near the vagina, and any pressure on the bladder can give you the feeling that you have to pee (see Illustration 21).

urethra (you-REE-thra)

If you press down on the vaginal walls, you may feel some lumps. This is because the lower part of your bowels lie just under the vagina, so you may be able to feel lumps of feces in the lower bowel.

If you slide your fingers more deeply into the vagina and press on the vaginal walls, you may notice that only about the first third of the vagina is very sensitive to your touch. The upper portion of the vagina is not as sensitive because it has fewer nerve endings.

The Cervix

At the top of the vagina, you may be able to feel a firm, round knob. This is the *cervix*, the lower part of the uterus that protrudes into the vagina (see Illustration 22). Like the vagina, the cervix grows larger during

cervix (SIR-vicks)

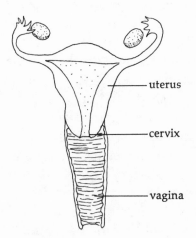

Illustration 22. The Cervix. The cervix is the lower portion of the uterus that protrudes into the vagina.

puberty. In grown women, it is about one to two inches in diameter.

It is not always easy to feel the cervix, since it is at the top of the vagina, but if you bear down as if you were making a bowel movement you should be able to feel it. It feels rather firm, like the tip of your nose. You may be able to feel a small depression or hole in the center of the cervix. This is the opening to the cervical canal, the tunnel that leads from the vagina into the uterus. This opening is called the os. It is no bigger around than the head of a kitchen match. Sperm pass through the os on their way to meet the ova. Menstrual blood passes through here when you are having your period. When a woman is having a baby, the cervical canal, like the vagina, stretches so the baby can pass through.

Your cervix and the walls of your vagina may feel wet, especially when you are sexually excited, for there are glands in here that make fluids that lubricate the vagina when we are sexually excited. Even if you are not feeling sexually excited, your vagina may feel rather wet. Like the skin on the outside of your body, the skin on the inside of the vagina is continually shedding old, dead cells. During puberty, the vaginal walls begin to shed cells at a faster rate than during childhood, and the vagina begins to make a small amount of fluid to wash these cells away. A year or two before your first menstrual period, you may start to notice a clear or milky-white, watery discharge from your vagina. It may leave a yellowish stain on your underpants when it dries. This discharge is made up of dead cells and fluid from the vaginal walls. This discharge is perfectly normal, just another one of the signs

os (OSZ)

that puberty is beginning. If, however, the discharge has a strong, offensive odor; causes itching or redness on your vulva; is brown, green, or a color other than clear or white; or if it changes from a watery liquid to a liquid with small, whitish chunks in it (rather like watery cottage cheese), then you may have an infection in your vagina. Such infections are not usually serious, but you should see a doctor so you can get them cleared up.

The Ovaries

The ovaries also get larger during puberty, but there is an even more dramatic change that takes place in the ovaries: It is during puberty that one of your ovaries will produce its first ripe ovum.

Unlike a male, who constantly makes a new supply of sperm in his body, a female is born with all the ova she will ever have. There are hundreds of thousands of ova in a girl's ovaries, but only eight or nine hundred of them will ever fully ripen.

The ripening process begins in the brain. When a girl is about eight years old, a part of her brain called the *pituitary* begins to send out substances called *hormones*. Hormones are made in one part of our bodies and travel to another part to act upon an organ there so that it develops or behaves in a particular way. Our bodies make hundreds of hormones. You could go crazy just trying to remember all their names. But in this book, we'll only bother with the hormones that are important in reproduction and puberty.

One of the hormones made by the pituitary during puberty is *FSH*, which is short for "follicle stimulating

pituitary (pih-TWO-eh-tear-ee)
hormones (HOR-moans)

hormone." During puberty, the FSH from the pituitary starts to get into the bloodstream and travels to the ovaries. It travels deep inside of the ovary where the tiny ova lie. Each ovum is encased in a tiny sac called a *follicle*. The follicle stimulating hormone, as its name implies, stimulates some of the follicles and their ova to grow and develop. It also causes the follicles to make yet another hormone called *estrogen* (see Illustration 23).

As a girl is going through puberty, her pituitary makes increasing amounts of FSH, which causes the follicles in the ovaries to make more and more estrogen. The estrogen also gets into the bloodstream and travels to other parts of the body. It is estrogen that causes many of the changes we notice during puberty. For example, estrogen travels to our breasts and causes the milk ducts and fat tissue to develop so that our breasts begin to swell and stand out. It causes fat tissue to develop on our hips, thighs, and buttocks, giving us a more curvy, womanly shape. Estrogen also causes pubic and other body hair to grow.

As the follicles in the ovary are developing and making increasing amounts of estrogen, they are also traveling toward the surface of the ovary. When they reach the surface, they press on the outer skin of the ovary, forming tiny bubbles that look like blisters.

Finally, when a girl is making a sufficient amount of estrogen, her pituitary gland slows down its production of FSH for a while and starts making another hormone called *LH*, or "luteinizing hormone." The LH travels to the ovary and causes one of the tiny bubbles on the

follicle (FOL-eh-kul)
estrogen (ES-tro-jen)
luteinizing (LOOT-in-eyes-ing)

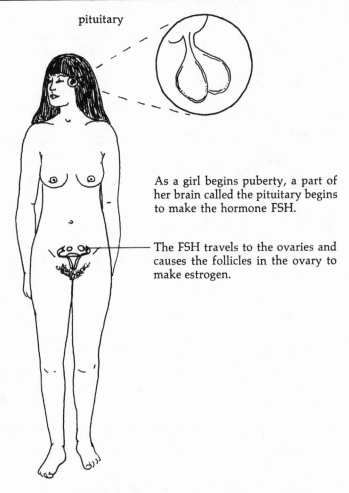

pituitary

As a girl begins puberty, a part of her brain called the pituitary begins to make the hormone FSH.

The FSH travels to the ovaries and causes the follicles in the ovary to make estrogen.

Illustration 23. Hormones. The estrogen that a girl's ovaries begin to make during puberty travels throughout her body, causing many changes, including the growth of pubic hair, swelling of the breasts, and development of fat tissue around her hips.

surface of the ovary to pop, and the ripe ovum bursts off the ovary. *Ovulation* is what we call this process of the ovum popping off the ovary (see Illustration 24).

ovulation (ahv-u-LAY-shun)

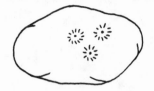

FSH from the pituitary causes some of the follicles in the ovary to develop and to make estrogen.

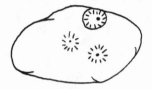

As more and more FSH reaches the ovaries, the follicles make increasing amounts of estrogen and move toward the surface of the ovary.

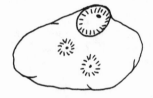

One of the follicles reaches the surface and presses on the outer skin of the ovary, forming a bubble.

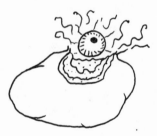

When a girl is making enough estrogen, the pituitary slows down its production of FSH and makes LH. The LH travels to the ovary, causing the follicle to burst and release its tiny ovum.

Illustration 24. Ovulation

Although some girls feel a slight twinge or a dull ache or even a strong pain when ovulation happens, most of us never feel the ovum popping off. A girl may ovulate for the first time when she is as young as eight or she may not ovulate until she is sixteen or older.

After ovulation, the fringed ends of the fallopian tube reach out to grasp the ovum and draw it into the tube.

The Fallopian Tubes

The fallopian tubes, through which ova travel on their way to the uterus, also grow longer and wider during puberty. But even in grown women, they are no thicker around than a strand of spaghetti. By the time we are grown women, each tube is about four inches long. The insides of the fallopian tubes are lined with tiny hairs, called *cilia*, which are attached to the muscles of the walls of the tubes. These muscles can contract and release, causing the tiny cilia to wave back and forth. It is this back-and-forth movement of the cilia that moves the ripe ovum down the length of the tube and into the uterus (see Illustration 25).

cilia (SIL-ee-uh)

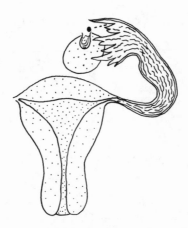

Illustration 25. The Ovum. The ovum travels through the fallopian tube to the uterus.

The Uterus

Like the other reproductive organs, the uterus also changes as we go through puberty. It too grows larger, but even in grown women it is only about the size of a clenched fist. The drawings in Illustration 26 are actual life-size drawings of the uterus and ovaries in a typical eleven-year-old girl and in a grown woman. Try tracing them, cutting them out, and holding them up to your own body. Doing this will help you to understand the size and location of these organs and how they change as you go through puberty.

As you can see from Illustration 20 at the beginning of this chapter, the uterus not only grows larger, it also changes position during puberty. In a young girl, the uterus is in an upright, almost vertical position, but as she grows older, it begins to lean forward, so it is tilted

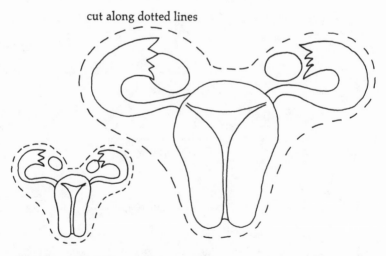

cut along dotted lines

Illustration 26. The Uterus and Ovaries. Approximate drawings of uterus, fallopian tubes, and ovaries in a typical eleven-year-old girl and a grown woman.

toward the bladder. This doesn't happen to all of us. Some women have what is called a tipped uterus (see Illustration 27), which means that the uterus has remained in its nearly upright position or has tipped in the other direction. It was once thought that having a tipped uterus might make it difficult for a woman to have a baby. All manner of backaches and problems were blamed on the tipped uterus. Doctors even performed operations to tip the uterus forward. We now

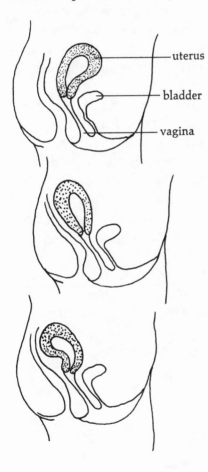

uterus

bladder

vagina

In most grown women, the uterus leans forward, toward the bladder.

But in some women, the uterus is in a more upright, vertical position.

In other women, the uterus is tipped backward, tilted away from the bladder.

Illustration 27. Tipped Uterus

know that having a tipped uterus has nothing to do with how likely you are to get pregnant or with any other sorts of problems.

The Endometrium

The lining of the uterus is called the *endometrium*. During childhood, it is very thin, but during puberty it too changes. When the ovaries begin to make enough estrogen, the lining starts to grow thick with new blood vessels and spongy, cushioning tissues. By the time the LH from the pituitary has caused the first ripe egg to pop off the ovary, the endometrium has doubled in thickness and is rich with blood.

After the ovum pops off the ovary, the endometrium undergoes yet another change. The LH from the pituitary that caused the follicle on the surface of the ovary to burst also causes the remnants of the burst follicle to turn a bright yellow color. The bright yellow leftover pieces of the burst follicle on the surface of the ovary are called the *corpus luteum* from the Latin words *corpus*, meaning "body," and *luteum*, meaning "yellow" (see Illustration 28).

The corpus luteum then begins to make another hormone. This hormone is called *progesterone*, and it travels to the uterus and causes the endometrium to grow still thicker and to make nourishing substances that can help a fertilized seed develop and grow into a baby.

If the ovum has been fertilized and the woman is

endometrium (en-doe-MEE-tree-um)
corpus (KORE-pus)
luteum (LOOT-ee-um)
progesterone (pro-JES-teh-rown)

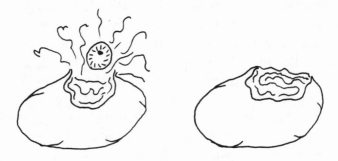

Illustration 28. Corpus Luteum. After the follicle containing the ovum has burst open, the remnants of the burst follicle turn bright yellow. These remnants are referred to as the corpus luteum.

going to have a baby, the corpus luteum keeps on making progesterone for a while, so that endometrium will continue to secrete the nourishment the baby will need. If the ovum hasn't been fertilized, the corpus luteum stops making progesterone and disintegrates within a few days. Without the help of the hormone progesterone, the lining of the uterus begins to break down. The spongy tissue and blood of the lining fall off the wall of the uterus, collect on the bottom of the uterus, and dribble through the cervical canal and out the os, into the vagina. (See Illustration 5 on page 33.) From there, the blood and tissues trickle down the vaginal walls and out the vaginal opening, and a girl has her menstrual period. The bleeding continues for a few days and then stops.

The Menstrual Cycle and Menopause

After a girl has had her first period, she continues ovulating (popping a ripe ovum off her ovary) and having her period (bleeding for a few days) about once a month for many, many years. This monthly process of ovaluating and menstruating is called the *menstrual cycle*. Although the menstrual cycle repeats itself for many years, it does not continue forever. Once a woman reaches a certain age, usually between forty-five and fifty-five, her ovaries stop producing a ripe ovum each month, and she no longer has her monthly bleeding period. Just as we have the word *puberty* for the time in a young woman's life when she first *starts* ovulating and menstruating, so we have a word for the time in an older woman's life when she *stops* ovulating and menstruating. This time in a woman's life is called *menopause*.

Menopause may happen very abruptly. A woman may have her period one month, then the next month she doesn't have her period and never has one again. Or it may happen gradually. A woman may skip one, two (or more) periods, and then have one or two (or more periods), skip some and then have her period again for a while, and so on, until she finally stops altogether.*

As a woman is going through menopause, her body is making less of the hormones estrogen and progesterone. Most women adjust to this change in their body chemistry with no problems. Some women have hot flashes, brief episodes in which their body heats up and they perspire profusely, as they are going through menopause. For most women, hot flashes, although bothersome, are not so severe that they need a doctor's care, but a few women have such severe and frequent

menopause (MEN-o-pause)

---

* Menopause is not the only reason women skip menstrual periods; see pages 151–53 for more details.

hot flashes that they need to seek medical care to help in controlling them.

Just as there are many myths and misconceptions about hymens and about masturbation, so there are many myths about menopause. Women going through menopause, or the "change of life," as it is sometimes called, supposedly are prone to fits of depression, anxiety, or crazy behavior. People used to think that a woman going through menopause would suddenly grow old, develop wrinkles, get fat, and feel less sexual desire. Today we know that menopause doesn't really cause any of these things. But there are many people who still have myths and misconceptions about menopause, so you may hear some of these things. If so, just ignore them.

But menopause is many years away for you, and you're probably more interested in learning about how menstruation works and about having your first period. We'll be talking about these things in the next chapter, but first we'd like to cover a couple of topics that inevitably come up in our "Everything You Ever Wanted to Know" question box when we talk about the reproductive organs.

Twins

When we talk about reproduction, about how babies are made, questions about twins inevitably come up. Twins can happen in one of two ways: Either there are two fertilized seeds, or there is one fertilized seed that has split into two (see Illustration 29).

Usually, a woman's ovaries only produce one ripe ovum a month. Sometimes, though, a woman will produce two ripe ova at the same time. If both of these ova are fertilized and plant themselves in the

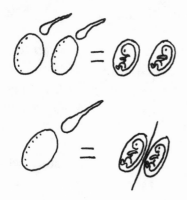

Sometimes a woman will produce two ripe ova the same month. If each of these ova is fertilized by sperm, the woman will have fraternal twins.

At other times, a sperm may fertilize a single ripe ovum. Then, after fertilization, the ovum splits into two, and the woman will have identical twins.

Illustration 29. Twins

uterus, the woman will have twins. Twins that grow from two separate ova, fertilized by two separate sperm, are called *fraternal twins*. They may both be boys or both girls, or one may be a boy and the other a girl. Even though they're born at the same time (one right after the other), they don't necessarily look alike.

The other type of twins are *identical twins*. Identical twins happen when the fertilized ovum and sperm split into two fertilized seeds shortly after fertilization has taken place. No one knows why this happens. Twins that come from the same egg and sperm look almost exactly alike and are always the same sex (either both are boys or both are girls).

Triplets (three babies), quadruplets (four), quintuplets (five), sextuplets (six), septuplets (seven), and octuplets (eight) happen less frequently than twins, and they are usually fraternal rather than identical.

We also get a lot of questions about Siamese twins. Siamese twins are identical twins who are born with their bodies attached to each other in some way. Siamese twins happen when the fertilized seed is splitting into two, making identical twins. For some unknown reason, the split is not complete and the babies develop so that some part of their bodies are joined together.

Identical twins are pretty rare. Identical Siamese twins are even more rare. When Siamese twins do happen, they may be joined together in any of a number of different ways. For instance, they may be joined at the shoulder, the arms, or the feet. When they are attached in such places, they are generally fairly easy to separate. A doctor can operate (usually shortly after the babies are born) and cut the babies apart. But sometimes it is not so easy. The babies may be joined at the head or at the chest in such a way that cutting them apart would kill them. In such cases, they simply have to grow up attached to each other (see Illustration 30).

Hermaphrodites

Another question that always comes up when we talk about male and female sex organs is whether a person can have both male and female sex organs. The answer is yes. People who have both male and female sex organs are called *hermaphrodites*.

Hermaphrodites have both testicles and ovaries on the inside of their bodies. On the outside, they may look a number of different ways. A hermaphrodite might, for example, have a penis, a man's body build, a beard, but have breasts like a woman. A hermaphrodite can also look like a woman with a curvy body shape, breasts, no beard, and have a penis instead of female genital organs. Or a hermaphrodite might have a vulva with inner and outer lips and a penis instead of a clitoris.

hermaphrodite (her-MAF-row-dite)

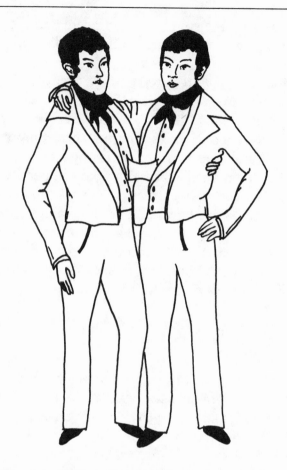

Illustrations 30. Siamese Twins. Perhaps the most famous Siamese twins, the Bunker brothers, were born in 1811. They were attached at the chest. They lived that way throughout their adult lives. If they had been born today, doctors would have been able to separate them.

Most of the time, it's obvious right from the moment of birth that a person is a hermaphrodite because of the way the genital organs look. But occasionally a hermaphrodite will have normal-looking genital organs at birth and throughout childhood, so everyone assumes the person is either male or female (depending on which kind of genital organs the hermaphrodite has). But, when puberty starts, it becomes obvious that this person is a hermaphrodite. For instance, a hermaphrodite who has normal-looking male sex organs during childhood may start to grow breasts during puberty. Or a hermaphrodite who has normal-looking female sex organs during childhood may develop a male body shape, grow a beard, and fail to start menstruating and to develop breasts.

When I explain to my class about hermaphrodites, I usually see a few kids gulping and looking very nervous and worried. The girls who haven't had their menstrual periods or whose breasts haven't begun developing start wondering if they really are females. If the other girls their age have started their periods and to develop breasts and they haven't, or if (like many girls) they've started to grow some dark hairs on their upper lips, then they start worrying, Oh, no, maybe I'm a hermaphrodite! Some of the boys usually look worried, too, especially if they've noticed their breasts swelling (many boys' breasts swell a bit as they are going through puberty).

I tell them not to worry. Hermaphrodites are usually mentally retarded, so if you're smart enough to go to school and to read this book, you don't need to worry about being a hermaphrodite.

But, enough of these more strange topics, let's move on to the menstrual cycle and having your first period.

CHAPTER 7

The Monthly Miracle: The Menstrual Cycle

Once a month, deep inside our bodies, the ovary begins, ever so slowly, to turn. The bubble on its surface contains the one ovum that has, for some mysterious reason, been chosen from all of the hundreds of thousands of ova to be released that month. The funnel-like opening at the end of the fallopian tube, lined with thousands of undulating cilia, turns to meet the ovary.

Suddenly, the bubble bursts. Triggered by a spurt of luteinizing hormone, the chemical messenger from the pituitary, the ovary contracts sharply and the ripe ovum bursts forth. The fringed ends of the fallopian tubes reach out like fingers to grasp the ripe ovum and draw it into the narrow tunnel of the tube. In a dream-like, slow-motion ballet, the tiny cilia caress the ripe ovum and gently move it along on its four-inch, four-day journey to the uterus.

As the ovum is moving through the tube toward the uterus, the lining of the uterus is preparing itself. The blood vessels in the area swell, flooding the uterus with a rich supply of blood to nourish the soft, spongy tissue of the uterine lining, which will cushion the ovum when it arrives. Glands in the uterus pour forth a banquet of nutrients that will nourish the developing ovum. The lining of the uterus has thickened to twice its normal depth—a luxuriously rich topsoil in which the ovum, if fertilized during the journey through the tube, will implant.

For the first three days after its arrival, the tiny ovum floats freely within the plush uterus. If fertilized, it will embed itself in the uterus on the seventh day. Meanwhile, on the surface of the ovary, the remnant of the burst bubble, the corpus luteum, which has turned a bright yellow after its explosive spasm, awaits a message from the uterus.

If in the upper reaches of the dark, narrow fallopian tube no sperm meets and fertilizes the ovum, the ovum will not implant in the lining of the uterus. Then the corpus luteum begins to disintegrate. The chemical messages it's been transmitting to the uterus via the hormone progesterone cease. The levels of progesterone in the bloodstream drop. Without the continued supply of progesterone from the corpus luteum, the swollen network of blood vessels shrinks, restricting the flow of blood to the lining. This deprives the newly grown tissues in the lining of their support and nourishment. Over a period of days, the lining falls away in small pieces. Within hours the now weakened blood vessels of the lining open, a few at a time. Each tiny vessel empties its droplets. More and more droplets are released and the flow of menstrual blood empties the uterus of the no-longer-needed tissues.

After some days of bleeding, the lining is emptied out and this process begins all over again. The uterine lining starts to grow rich and thick again, and more ova begin to move toward the surface of the ovary. Another ovum is released at ovulation, and if the woman is not going to have a baby, then her period begins again about two weeks after ovulation.

The Menstrual Cycle

The time from the first day of bleeding of one menstrual period to the first day of bleeding of the next period—the menstrual cycle—takes about a month. The menstrual cycle may last for anywhere from twenty-one to thirty-five days. The average is about twenty-eight days. But there are very few women who actually have their periods regularly, every twenty-eight days, like clockwork, throughout their entire lives. Most of us are somewhat more irregular than this. For example, in the last year, my periods went like this: My first three periods of the year were very regular. I began to bleed once every twenty-nine days, and the bleeding lasted for five days each time. My fourth period came twenty-seven days after my third and lasted for only four days. Then I didn't have a period again for thirty days, and when I did have it, it lasted for six days. My next period came thirty-one days later and lasted for five days. Then I started having my periods more regularly again, once every twenty-nine days, and I bled for five days each time.

Each of us has her own pattern. Some are more regular than others. We may be very regular and suddenly get irregular, as one woman explained:

> I was very regular when I was younger. I could set my watch by it, once every twenty-six days. Then, when I

turned thirty, I got real irregular—once every twenty-two days, once every twenty-six, once every thirty. Now, I'm more regular again.

On the other hand, some women are very irregular and then suddenly their periods start to get regular. No one is exactly sure why some women are regular and others irregular or why our patterns may change. But we do know that traveling, emotional ups and downs, illness, and such things can affect our menstrual periods, making them start earlier or later than usual. There is an old-wives' tale that says that women who live together, who spend a lot of time with each other, or who are close friends tend to have their periods around the same time, which might also account for why our patterns change. "That's certainly true for me," one woman told us:

> I've always menstruated about the same time as the other women I'm around. When I lived at home, my sisters and I always had our periods together at the beginning of each month. When I went away to college, I found that my periods changed. I started menstruating around the middle of the month, same as my roommates.

As it turns out, this old-wives' tale may have a great deal of truth to it. Scientific studies have shown that women who are close do often have their periods around the same time.

Young women who've just started having their periods are particularly likely to have irregular periods. It takes a while for our bodies to adjust to menstruating. You may have your first period and not have another one for six months. Or you may have your second period two weeks after your first one. It often takes two or three years to develop anything near a regular pattern, and some of us never do get very regular.

Length of Your Period/Amount and Type of Blood Flow

Your period may last anywhere from two to seven days. The average is about five days. Some of your periods may last longer than others, so one month you may bleed for only two or three days, and the next time you may bleed for five or six days. Or you may be one of those women who bleeds for exactly five days each time. Here again, each of us has our own individual pattern, and our patterns may change over the course of our lives.

Although it may seem as if a lot of blood comes out of the uterus, it isn't really that much. The amount of blood may vary from one tablespoon to one cup. Women have different patterns in this too. Some of us always have heavy periods, about eight tablespoons each time; others always have light periods, only one tablespoon each time. Still others vary between having heavy and light periods.

Some of us tend to bleed most heavily on the first day or two, gradually trickling off until there is only a light flow of blood on the last day. Others start off lightly on the first day, then get heavier. Still others will bleed for a number of days and stop or slow down to only a trickle for a day or so, then bleed more heavily again. All these patterns, or any combination of these patterns, is normal.

The blood and tissue that comprise the menstrual flow may be thin and watery, or the flow may have thick clumps called clots. You may be more apt to notice clots in the morning when you get up, for the blood has been pooling and congealing in the top of the vagina while you've been lying down asleep.

The blood may be bright red to brown in color. It is

especially likely to be brownish at the very beginning or toward the end of your period. Blood tends to turn brown the longer it sits. If your blood has been slow in moving out of your body, it may take on a brownish color.

The Four Phases

Regardless of whether your periods usually come every twenty-one days or every thirty-five days, whether they're regular or irregular, light or heavy, the menstrual cycle works in essentially the same way in all of us. The menstrual cycle can be divided into four parts, or phases.

PHASE 1

The first phase of the menstrual cycle is the bleeding phase, when you are actually having your period. During this phase, the uterine lining is breaking down and being shed. We call the first day of bleeding Day 1 of your menstrual cycle. As we said, the bleeding phase may last for one to seven days, but it usually lasts about five days. So, for purposes of this discussion, we'll call Day 1 to Day 5 the first, or bleeding, phase of the cycle (see Illustration 31).

PHASE 2

During this phase, the pituitary gland is making FSH, which causes the follicles in the ovary to make estrogen and to move toward the surface of the ovary. The estrogen also causes the lining of the uterus to develop new blood passageways and spongy tissues to cushion them.

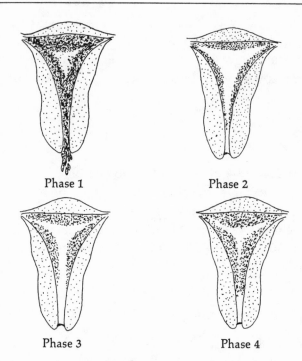

Phase 1

Phase 2

Phase 3

Phase 4

Illustration 31. The Uterus in the Four Stages of the Menstrual Cycle

In a woman with a twenty-eight-day cycle who bleeds for five days, this phase would start on about Day 6 and would continue until Day 13 or so. Of course, if your cycle is longer or shorter than twenty-eight days, this phase may be longer or shorter.

PHASE 3

By the end of Phase 2, the ovaries are making enough estrogen so that the pituitary gland slows down its production of FSH and releases a spurt of LH. The LH travels to the ovary and causes the bubble on the surface of the ovary that contains the ripe ovum to pop. This phase is, then, the ovulation phase, the phase in which the ripe egg is released from the ovary.

Generally, the ovaries only produce one ripe ovum during each menstrual cycle. Scientists believe that the ovaries take turns. During one cycle, the right ovary ovulates, and during the following cycle, the left ovary does. If a woman only has one ovary, either because she was born with only one or one has been removed because it was diseased, then the remaining ovary takes over and produces a ripe ovum each month.

Most women don't feel anything when the bubble bursts and the ripe ovum pops off the ovary; however, some women do know when they are ovulating because they feel a cramp or a pain. Some women have a dull achy feeling for a day or so around the time they are ovulating. Others have a sudden sharp pain that passes very quickly; still others experience just a mild twinge that is hardly noticeable. But for most of us ovulation happens without our being aware of it.

In a woman with a twenty-eight-day cycle, ovulation usually occurs on Day 14; however, it may happen one or two days earlier or later than this—that is, anywhere from Day 12 to Day 16.

Most books that describe the menstrual cycle talk about a twenty-eight-day cycle and explain that ovulation occurs about halfway through the cycle, on Day 14. Women who have longer or shorter cycles often assume that they too will ovulate at the halfway point of their cycles. Thus, many women think that ovulation would occur halfway through a thirty-two-day cycle, on about Day 16, or halfway in a twenty-two-day cycle, on Day 11. This is not true. Ovulation occurs about fourteen days (give or take one or two days either way) before the first day of bleeding of the next period. So, if a woman has a thirty-two-day cycle, she probably ovulates around Day 18 (32 — 14 = 18), and if she has a twenty-two-day cycle, she probably ovulates around Day 8 (22 — 14 = 8).

A woman can get pregnant only during the ovulation phase of her menstrual cycle, when her ovary has just recently released the ripe ovum. It would be nice if we could predict exactly when a woman is going to ovulate. That way, a woman who wanted to get pregnant could have sexual intercourse at a time when her chances of getting pregnant are highest, and a woman who didn't want to get pregnant could avoid having intercourse at this time. But it doesn't work that way. One month a woman might have a twenty-eight-day cycle so she'd ovulate around Day 14. But the next month she might have a thirty-five-day cycle, so she'd probably ovulate around Day 21. The following cycle might only be twenty-one days long, so she'd ovulate around Day 7.

Attempting to prevent pregnancy by trying to figure out when you are going to ovulate and avoiding sex at that time doesn't work very well. This method of preventing pregnancy, this method of birth control, is referred to as the *rhythm method.* There are other, more effective methods of birth control. If you are interested in learning more about birth control, there are a number of excellent books that talk about it (see "For Further Reading"). You might want to talk to your mother and other women to find out what, if any, method of birth control they use. If you are just starting to menstruate, you probably won't be having intercourse, so you won't need to concern yourself with birth control for a number of years. But it's a good idea to start learning about these things when you are young, so that when you do begin to have sexual intercourse, you are well informed.

PHASE 4

As this phase begins, the ripe ovum is in the fallopian tube, traveling toward the uterus. The corpus luteum, the remnants of the burst follicle on the surface of the ovary, has turned a bright yellow color and is making progesterone. The progesterone is causing the lining of the uterus to get even thicker and to secrete nutrients.

If a sperm manages to make its way into the fallopian tube at this time, there's a good chance that fertilization will take place. The sperm penetrates the outer shell of the ovum, and the fertilized seed then travels to the uterus. It plants itself in the rich uterine lining.

If fertilization takes place, the corpus luteum continues to produce progesterone for some time so that the uterine lining will provide nutrients to nourish the fertilized ovum. But most of the time fertilization doesn't happen. The ovum disintegrates. Because fertilization hasn't happened, the corpus luteum also disintegrates and stops producing progesterone.

At this point in the menstrual cycle there is very little estrogen and very little progesterone being made in our bodies, so the lining of the uterus starts to break down and is shed. As the lining is being shed, the pituitary starts making more FSH. In turn, the ovaries start making more estrogen. As soon as the lining is shed, a new lining begins to thicken, and the menstrual cycle starts all over again.

In a woman with a twenty-eight-day cycle, Phase 4 would run from about Day 15 (right after ovulation) until Day 28. On the twenty-ninth day, the bleeding would start again and thus would be Day 1 of the next cycle.

SUMMARY OF THE FOUR PHASES OF THE MENSTRUAL CYCLE

Phase 1
- The uterine lining is being shed; the woman is having her period.
- The pituitary and the ovaries are only making small amounts of hormones.

Phase 2
- The pituitary is making FSH.
- The ovaries are making estrogen.
- The follicles in the ovary are moving toward the surface of the ovary.
- The uterine lining is starting to thicken.

Phase 3
- The pituitary releases a spurt of LH.
- The ripe ovum bursts from the ovary and moves into the fallopian tube.

Phase 4
- The remnants of the burst follicle become the corpus luteum and begin to make progesterone.
- The progesterone makes the uterine lining grow even thicker.
- If fertilization occurs, the corpus luteum keeps making progesterone; if not, the corpus luteum disintegrates.
- Without progesterone from the corpus luteum, the uterine lining breaks down and is shed. The first day of bleeding is Day 1 of the next cycle.

Menstruation—When?

The girls in my class always want to know, "When will I have my first period?" Unfortunately, I can't answer that question. Each of us has our own timetable. No one can say exactly when it will happen, but I *can* give you an idea. A girl may have her first period any time between her eighth and sixteenth birthdays. But very few girls have their periods when they are as young as eight, and the vast majority have theirs before they are sixteen. In fact, most girls have their periods between their eleventh and fourteenth birthdays. Still, there are plenty of girls who have their periods when they are only eight or nine and plenty who don't have theirs until fifteen or sixteen. If you reach the age of sixteen and have not started menstruating, it's a good idea to see a gynecologist, a doctor who specializes in women's health care. Not menstruating by the age of sixteen isn't necessarily a sign that there's something wrong. There have been cases of perfectly normal girls who didn't start to menstruate until their twenties, but it's a good idea to see a doctor to rule out the possibility that you have a medical problem that is keeping you from menstruating.

Even though it's impossible to say exactly when any particular girl will have her first period, there are some clues. One thing that may give you a clue as to when you'll start is when your mother started. Daughters often have their first periods around the same age that their mothers did. This is not a hard-and-fast rule, but it is at least a clue. See if your mom can remember exactly when she started.

You might want to use the chart on page 127 to keep track of your progress through puberty. Perhaps keeping a chart like this is something you and your mom, a girlfriend, or another person you feel close to could do together, and it might be fun to share this chart with your daughter if someday you become the mother of a girl.

Start by filling in the first section of the chart. Every three months or so fill in a new section. (Make more chart pages as you need them.) Begin by writing in the date and recording your height and weight. If you have not yet begun your growth spurt, you may notice a dramatic increase in your height and weight as time passes and you fill in more sections on the chart. If your growth spurt has already started, you'll probably notice a more gradual increase in your height and weight.

On the next line, where it says "Stage of Pubic Hair Development," write the numeral 1, 2, 3, 4, or 5 to indicate which stage of pubic hair development you are in now. It might be helpful to turn back to Illustration 9, on page 46, which shows the five stages of pubic hair development. If you don't have any pubic hairs at all, you would write the numeral 1 on that line of the chart. If you have at least a few pubic hairs, you would write the numeral 2 there. If your pubic hair looks more like the drawing of Stage 3, write a 3, and so on. If you are between stages, you might want to write something like "between Stage 2 and 3" or "between Stage 3 and 4."

On the next line, the one that says "Stage of Breast Development," write the stage you are closest to right now. It might be helpful to look at Illustration 12 on page 61. Again, if you're between stages, you might want to make a note of this.

If you notice other changes, for example, underarm hair, dark hair on your arms and legs, more perspiration, pimples, a change in the appearance of your vulva, a vaginal discharge—note these things on your chart in the space after the words "Other Changes." Any time you notice something new, fill in another section of the chart, even if it hasn't been three months since your last entry. Of course, when you first menstruate, mark that on the chart too!

MY PUBERTY CHART

Date:
Height: Weight:
Stage of Pubic Hair
   Development:
Stage of Breast
   Development:
Other Changes:

Date:
Height: Weight:
Stage of Pubic Hair
   Development:
Stage of Breast
   Development:
Other Changes:

Date:
Height: Weight:
Stage of Pubic Hair
   Development:
Stage of Breast
   Development:
Other Changes:

Date:
Height: Weight:
Stage of Pubic Hair
   Development:
Stage of Breast
   Development:
Other Changes:

Date:
Height: Weight:
Stage of Pubic Hair
   Development:
Stage of Breast
   Development:
Other Changes:

Date:
Height: Weight:
Stage of Pubic Hair
   Development:
Stage of Breast
   Development:
Other Changes:

Date:
Height: Weight:
Stage of Pubic Hair
   Development:
Stage of Breast
   Development:
Other Changes:

Date:
Height: Weight:
Stage of Pubic Hair
   Development:
Stage of Breast
   Development:
Other Changes:

Keeping a chart like this of the stages of pubic hair and breast development can give you some idea of when you'll start to menstruate. Doctors have studied groups of girls going through puberty to see what stages of breast and pubic development girls were in when they started to menstruate. The following table shows the results of these studies.

WHEN GIRLS STARTED TO MENSTRUATE

Stage	Percentage* of girls who started to menstruate in each stage of breast development	Percentage* of girls who started to menstruate in each stage of pubic hair hair growth
1	0%	1%
2	1%	4%
3	26%	19%
4	62%	63%
5	11%	14%

* Percentage means part of 100. If we say 62 percent of all girls menstruate when they are in breast Stage 4, we mean that of a group of 100 girls, 62 of them will have their first period while they are in Stage 4 of breast development.

As you can see from this table, most girls (62 percent) start to menstruate when they are in Stage 4 of breast development. Also, most girls (63 percent) have their first periods in Stage 4 of pubic hair development. So if your puberty chart shows you've reached Stage 4 of breast and pubic hair development, you can expect to start menstruating in the near future. However, as you can also see from the table, 11 percent of girls don't have their periods until Stage 5 of breast development and 14 percent don't start until Stage 5 of pubic hair development. Moreover, a fair number of girls, 26 percent, start their periods while they are in breast Stage 3, and 19 percent start while they are in pubic hair Stage 3.

None of the girls studied started to menstruate while they were in breast Stage 1 and only 1 percent (1 out of 100) started in pubic hair Stage 1. So if you are still in Stage 1, you probably won't start menstruating until you've moved to a more advanced stage of breast and pubic hair development.

Breast development and pubic hair development don't always go together. So you may be in one stage of breast development and in another stage of pubic hair development. For example, one of the girls in our class had her first period when she was in Stage 4 of breast development and Stage 3 of pubic hair development.

Another question that often comes up in our classes is, "How long does it take to go through the various stages?" Again it's hard to answer this question exactly, but we do know how long most girls take to go through them.

LENGTH OF TIME THAT GIRLS REMAIN IN VARIOUS STAGES

Stage	Most Girls	95 Percent of All Girls
Breast Stage 2	About 11 months	About 2½ to 12 months
Breast Stage 3	About 11 months	About 4 to 26 months
Breast Stage 4	24 months	About 1 month to 7 years
Pubic Hair Stage 2	About 7 months	About 2½ to 15½ months
Pubic Hair Stage 3	6 months	About 2½ to 11 months
Pubic Hair Stage 4	About 15½ months	About 7 to 29 months

As you can see, most girls spend about eleven months in Stage 2 of breast development. In other words, it takes eleven months to get from the beginning of Stage 2 to the beginning of Stage 3. But that's only most girls. Some girls take as little as two-and-one-half months and some as long as twelve months. There are a few girls (about 5 percent) who will take either a shorter or longer time than this.

Likewise, reading across the second line of the table will tell you that most girls spend about eleven months in breast Stage 3. Some girls take as little as one month to get through Stage 3 and some take as many as twenty-six months. Ninety-five percent of us will take somewhere between one and twenty-six months; most of us will take about eleven months.

Your First Period

These charts and tables are fun to fool around with and they can give you some idea of when you can expect to start menstruating, but no one can predict the exact day of your first period and this worries many girls.

"What'll I do if it happens when I'm at school?" is a question that often comes up in my classes. Luckily, there are usually some girls in my classes who've already started to menstruate and can share their experiences with the other girls. Here's what one of them had to say:

> I got my first period during history class. I wasn't sure if it was happening, but I sort of knew. So I raised my hand and said I had to go to the bathroom. Sure enough, there was blood on my underpants. Luckily, I had my purse with some change in it, so I got a sanitary napkin out of the machine and pinned it to my underpants and just went back to class.

Sanitary napkins are pads of soft cotton that are used to absorb the menstrual flow. This girl was lucky. There was a napkin machine in the girl's room and she had some change with her. Another girl wasn't so lucky:

> I got my period at school, too. I kinda knew right away what it was, but I went to the bathroom to check. There weren't any napkins in the machine, so I just wadded up some toilet paper and went to the nurse's office. She was real nice and gave me a clean pair of underpants and a napkin.

A number of girls said that they'd gone to the school nurse, to their gym teachers, to the secretary in the school office, or to a woman teacher for a sanitary napkin. If their underpants were bloody, sometimes the nurse or whoever had a spare pair. At other times, they'd just ignored the blood or they'd just rinsed their pants out with cold water and put them on while they were still damp or waited until they dried. Other girls said they'd gone to a telephone and called their moms who'd come to school with clean pants and napkins.

One girl told us that she'd been prepared:

> I knew I was getting old enough, so at the beginning of seventh grade, I put a sanitary napkin in my purse in those special carrying cases they give you. And I just kept it there so I'd be ready. The school I was going to didn't have a school nurse, and the napkin machines were always broken or empty. I didn't want to have to go into the office and say I was having my period and needed a napkin. There were always a lot of people in there. I would have been so embarrassed.

Another girl told us that she, too, had been prepared:

> I had that napkin in my purse for almost a year. I thought I was so smart—being ready and all.
>
> Then I'm walking down the hall one day and my girl friend says, "Hey, you got blood on your skirt." I almost died. "Stand in back of me," I said, and she walked down the hall kind of right behind me, so no one could see. I got my coat out of my locker and put it on and went to the office. I told the secretary I was sick and had to go home.

Most girls notice a feeling of wetness before the blood soaks through their underpants and onto their clothes. And most girls don't bleed enough right at first to have it show through on their clothes. But some girls had embarrassing stories to tell about how the blood had soaked through their clothes, making a spot. If you're feeling worried about your first period, why not talk it over with your mom or someone else who might have some helpful hints. Finding out what has happened to other people or just talking about your worries can help a lot.

Sanitary Napkins, Tampons, and Sponges

You can have your period any time, night or day, at home, at school, or anywhere you happen to be. Regardless of where or when it happens, you'll want to have some way of absorbing the menstrual flow.

In the past, women have used everything from grass to soft cloths and sponges to catch their menstrual flow. Nowadays, we have all sorts of menstrual products, so many that it may be hard to choose which ones you want to use. You might ask your mom or another woman which she prefers and why. You can also try the various products yourself until you hit on the ones you like best.

SANITARY NAPKINS OR PADS

Sanitary napkins come in different sizes and thicknesses and can be bought in supermarkets and drugstores. They are made of layers of soft cotton. Most of them have a piece of plastic lining to prevent the blood from soaking through the pad (see Illustration 32).

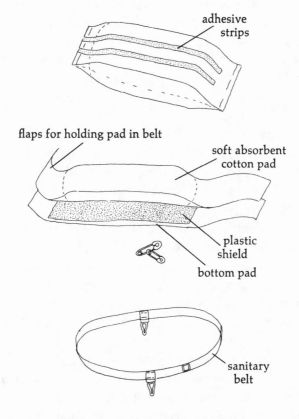

Illustration 32. Sanitary Napkins

Some sanitary napkins are made to be worn with a belt. The napkin fits to the belt, which is worn around the waist. You can also pin the napkin to your underpants with safety pins. Some napkins are made so that you don't need pins or a belt. They have a strip of sticky adhesive on the underside. The adhesive is covered by a strip of glossy paper. You remove the strip of paper and press the napkin into your underpants. The adhesive will hold the napkin in place.

If you have a heavy menstrual flow, you may need to use the thickest pads, at least on the days you are flowing heavily. If your flow is lighter, you may want to use one of the thinner pads, which are not as bulky. There are also very thin pads that some girls use on the last day or so of their period if they only have a small amount of blood.

Wearing a pad for the first time can feel rather strange, especially the thick ones. Even though it may feel as if everyone can see that you're wearing a pad, it really doesn't show. Check yourself out in the mirror and you'll see—the pad really isn't visible.

Sanitary napkins should be changed every three or four hours to avoid soaking through the pad. It's a good idea to change them frequently, even if you have a very light flow and don't have to worry about soaking through the pad. Menstrual blood itself is perfectly clean and odorless, but once it comes in contact with the germs in the vagina and in the air, it does develop an odor, because germs grow very rapidly in the rich blood. These germs aren't necessarily harmful, but they can cause an unpleasant odor. By changing your pad frequently, you won't give the germs and odor a chance to develop.

Used napkins should be put in a wastebasket or trashcan. Don't flush them down the toilet, as they will clog the plumbing. Public bathrooms often have special disposal containers for sanitary napkins right in the toilet stall. If there isn't one and you don't want to come waltzing out of the stall in front of everyone with a bloody napkin in your hand, fold the napkin in half and wrap it in toilet paper. Then, when you leave the stall, just toss it in the nearest trashcan. It's a good idea to wrap them up like this even when you're at home, for it will cut down on odor from the pad.

TAMPONS

Another way of catching the menstrual flow is to use a tampon. Women have been using tampons since the dawn of time. They made small rolls of absorbent grass or cloth and put the roll inside the vagina to absorb the blood. Nowadays, we have tampons made of absorbent cotton that usually have a string attached to the end so they can be easily removed. Most tampons come in an applicator to make it easier to insert the tampon into the vagina.

The girls in my class usually have a lot of questions about tampons. First of all, they want to know if a tampon can "go up inside you." The answer is no. The tampon goes through the vaginal opening, into the vagina, but it can't get up into the uterus. The passageway between the vagina and uterus, the cervical canal, is too small. The opening to the cervical canal, the cervical os, is no bigger around than the head of a matchstick. It's simply not possible for a tampon to get into the uterus.

The girls in my class also want to know whether a tampon can "get lost" in the vagina, usually because they've heard some story about a woman who had to go to the doctor because her tampon "got lost." A tampon can't really get lost in the vagina, but what can happen is that the string that is attached to the end of the tampon may get drawn up into the vagina, or the tampon may get so far into the vagina that the woman can't feel the string and thinks it's lost. If this should happen to you, relax—it's a simple matter to get it back out again. Just reach your fingers up inside your vagina and pull the tampon out. If it's way up inside there, you may have to squat or bear down as if you were making a bowel movement. This will push the tampon down lower so you can reach it. Most of the time, the tampon string dangles out of the vaginal opening and you just pull gently on the string to remove the tampon.

Girls also want to know whether a virgin, a person who has never had sexual intercourse, can use a tampon. The answer is yes. A girl can use a tampon regardless of her age and whether or not she's a virgin. It may be more difficult to use a tampon if you're young or if you only have small openings in your hymen. But your vaginal opening and your hymen are stretchy. If you have trouble getting the tampon in, try using your finger gently to stretch the opening. After a couple of months of gently stretching yourself a few times a week, you should be able to get the tampon in.

The girls in my class always want to know in exact detail how to get the tampon in. Since the instructions that come with most tampons are not very detailed, we always spend some time talking about how to insert a tampon.

Some women like to insert their tampons while they are standing up; others do it lying down; still others do it in a sitting position. Regardless of which position you use, it helps if you remember that the vagina doesn't go straight up and down, but angles toward the small of the back. If you don't insert the tampon at a slight angle, it's going to hit against the vaginal walls and will be much harder to insert.

Make sure, too, that you're using the right size tampon. Tampons, which can also be purchased in supermarkets and drugstores, come in three or four sizes. The small size may be called a regular or junior size and the largest is called a super. If you're just starting out, you will want the smallest, thinnest tampon as it will be easier to insert.

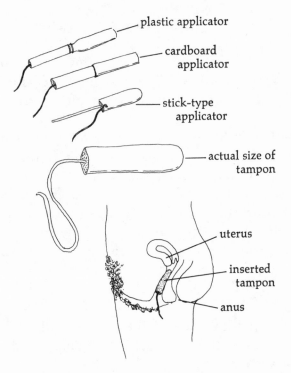

plastic applicator

cardboard applicator

stick-type applicator

actual size of tampon

uterus

inserted tampon

anus

Illustration 33. Tampons

If you're using a tampon with an applicator, spend a few minutes fooling around with one of the applicators so you'll know how it works. If your vaginal opening is dry, you might want to lubricate the tampon with a little saliva, petroleum jelly, or K-Y Jelly. Don't use hand or body lotions or face creams to lubricate the tampon; they may contain chemicals that could irritate your vulva and vagina.

It's important to relax because if you are tense, your muscles will tighten up and your vaginal opening will contract.

Be sure to remove the outer wrapping, then gently push the end of the tampon and applicator into your vagina to a depth of one-half to one inch. You may have to hold one portion of the applicator while you push on the plunger of the applicator. Some tampons come on a stick. You push the tampon up into the vagina with the stick. Others don't have any applicator at all; you just push the tampon up inside with your finger.

Now here's the part they never tell you in the instructions. If you don't push the tampon in far enough, it's going to feel uncomfortable. If you put a finger inside your vagina and tighten the muscles in the area by pulling in and up, you'll feel the muscles just inside your vaginal opening tighten. You'll want to get the tampon up above the point where those muscles tighten. Otherwise, the tampon is caught between the muscles and it will feel uncomfortable. If a tampon is inserted properly, you won't be able to feel it once it's in place. And there is no danger of the tampon falling out because the muscles just inside the vaginal opening will prevent it from slipping out.

If it hurts to insert the tampon, then use a sanitary napkin and try gently stretching your opening with your finger as we explained above. Then try a tampon again.

Like napkins, tampons should be changed every three or four hours. The tampon itself can be flushed down the toilet, but the applicator should be thrown in a wastecan as it could clog the toilet.

Tampons are so comfortable to wear that women sometimes forget they're there and may neglect to remove the last one at the end of their periods. This will eventually cause a foul odor and maybe a discharge, but after you remove the forgotten tampon, this should clear up.

SPONGES

Some women use sponges to catch the menstrual flow (see Illustration 34). The advantage of the sponge is that it can be taken out and rinsed clean and reused. I have several friends who use sponges and think they're the greatest thing in the world. I've tried them, and to tell you the truth, I didn't think they were so great. They tended to "leak" blood, but what really bothered me was that it seemed impossible to rinse the blood completely out of the sponge. If you decide to try sponges (which can usually be purchased at health food stores), be sure to rinse the blood out completely, and it might be wise to boil the sponge to get rid of other infection-causing germs.

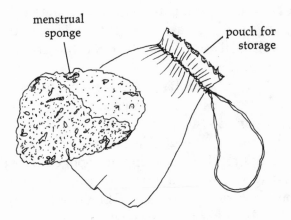

Illustration 34. Menstrual Sponge

TOXIC SHOCK SYNDROME

While we're on the subject of napkins, tampons, and sponges, we should probably mention *toxic shock syndrome* (TSS for short), which is a disease that has been associated with the use of tampons, napkins, and menstrual sponges. Most of the people who've gotten TSS have been women under the age of thirty who were having their periods at the time that they got the disease and who were using tampons or, less frequently, menstrual sponges or napkins. But males and younger and older females have also gotten TSS, as well as women who weren't menstruating at the time they came down with the disease.

TSS is an infection. When it is the result of using tampons, it starts in the vagina. It is caused by a germ that makes a poison or toxin that gets into the bloodstream. The disease usually starts with a sudden fever, vomiting, and diarrhea. Sometimes there is an accompanying headache, sore throat, or achy muscles. Within forty-eight hours, there may be a dramatic drop in blood pressure so that the person becomes very weak and groggy. A red rash that peels like sunburn may develop. The disease is rarely fatal, but some women have died of TSS.

No one is certain what tampons have to do with the disease, but most of the women who've gotten it were using tampons at the time. The majority were using a particular brand, the RELY tampon. But some were using other brands or napkins or sponges. The disease was first widely noticed about the time that the RELY tampon came on the market. RELY contained a new, superabsorbent fiber, and proved very popular.

Some of the researchers studying TSS think that

these superabsorbent fibers are the source of the problem. One theory is that because the superabsorbent fibers can soak up so much blood, women don't change them as often. Thus, the blood stays in the vagina longer. Blood, as we mentioned, can be a breeding ground for germs. If a woman happens to have a TSS-causing germ in her vagina and the tampon is left in the vagina long enough, the germs can multiply and make enough poison so that the woman becomes ill. Other researchers feel that the roughness of these tiny superabsorbent fibers also contributes to TSS by causing microscopic scratches on the inside of the vagina. They feel that the poisons get into the bloodstream through these scratches.

When the news about TSS first came out, many women stopped using tampons. But because sanitary napkins are more bulky, can cause chafing, are more likely to have an odor, and are so much less comfortable, many women went back to tampons. TSS is a rare disease, affecting only about six in every hundred thousand women, so if you want to use tampons, you probably aren't taking a very big risk.

If you do use tampons, change your tampon every three or four hours. Always change it before you go to bed and first thing when you wake up, or better yet, use a sanitary napkin at night. If you do develop a sudden fever (over 102°) and are vomiting, remove the tampon and see your doctor right away.

Is It All Right To . . .?

The girls in my class always have questions about whether it is okay to do certain things while they're having their periods: Is it all right to take a bath or a shower? To wash my hair? To go horseback riding? To take a gym class? To have sexual intercourse? To drink cold drinks or eat cold food?

The answer to all these questions is yes. You can do anything you'd do at any other time of the month. Of course, if you're going swimming during your menstrual period, you'll want to use a tampon instead of a sanitary napkin.

You may have heard that you shouldn't shower or bathe during your period, but this simply isn't true. In fact, you are apt to perspire more heavily while you're menstruating, so a daily shower or bath may be especially important. You may have heard that cold food or drinks or strenuous exercise would cause a heavier flow, cause your period to last longer, or cause you to have cramps. Again, none of this is true. In fact, exercise can sometimes help to relieve cramps.

Douching

Some women like to douche at the end of their menstrual period. Douching is a way of cleaning the vagina by flushing it out. Many doctors don't think douching is a very good idea. For one thing, it's not really necessary. Your vaginal walls secrete fluids that rinse your vagina and keep it clean naturally. Also, there is a slight chance of causing an infection. Still, some women like to douche because it makes them feel cleaner.

You can douche using a quart of water mixed with two tablespoons of white vinegar. Or you can buy one of the douche mixes that are sold in markets and drugstores; however, some of these can be irritating to the vagina. There are two types of douches, the bag type and the syringe type (see Illustration 35). The syringe

douching (DOOSH-ing)

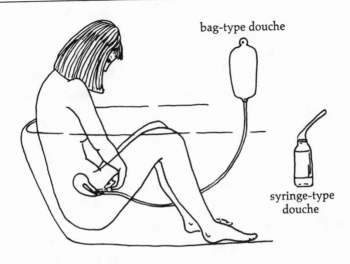

bag-type douche

syringe-type
douche

Illustration 35. Douching

has a bulb on the end, and you squeeze the bulb to push
the douche solution up into the vagina. Nowadays there
are disposable syringe douches that come prefilled with
douche solution or with vinegar and water. The bag
type, which looks like a hot-water bottle with a tube
coming out the end, is probably more effective than the
syringe type.

The bag type has a nozzle on the end of the tube that
is inserted into the vagina after the bag has been filled
with a douche solution. The woman sits in the bathtub,
inserts the nozzle, and holds the bag about a foot above
her hips. Releasing a clip on the hose allows the douche
solution to run from the bag, down into the tube, and
out the nozzle into the vagina. The solution then flushes
out the vagina and dribbles back out the vaginal opening. The higher above the hips the bag is, the more
forceful the flow of the douche solution into the vagina.
But too much pressure could force germs from the
vagina up into the sterile uterus, causing infection, so
keep the bag no more than a foot or so above your hips.

The douche bag should be washed with soap and water before and after each use. Douching equipment should not be shared, because infection could be transmitted this way. Before each use, check the nozzle for cracks that could injure your vagina tissues or harbor infection.

Cramps

Almost every woman has cramps at some time or other in her life. They may happen before or during menstrual periods. The cramps may be just a mild achy feeling, or they may be sharp and severe. Most women only have mild cramps, and they only have them once in a while. A few women get very severe cramps each and every time they menstruate.

No one knows why women have menstrual cramps, but there are a number of theories. One theory holds that cramps happen because the uterus contracts rhythmically while we're having our periods to help expel the menstrual blood. Women who are particularly sensitive may feel these contractions as cramps. Another theory holds that cramps are caused by excessive amounts of hormones called *prostaglandins*. Prostaglandins help the uterus contract, and women who have problems with cramps often have more prostaglandins in their bodies than women who aren't troubled by cramps.

The theories go on and on. One particularly popular theory says that cramps are "all in your head." This theory is often held by doctors, who are mostly men, so maybe it's not surprising that they think "it's all in

prostaglandins (PROST-uh-glan-dins)

your head." There are plenty of women who believe this theory too, but if you've ever had severe menstrual cramps, you know it's not in your head—it's in your belly—and it hurts.

If you are troubled by cramps, there are some home remedies you can try. Exercises like the ones in Illustration 36 have proven helpful for many women.

Masturbating until you have an orgasm may be helpful, for after you have an orgasm, the blood vessels in the area are less congested, and blood flows more freely. Likewise, massaging your lower abdomen or using a heating pad or hot-water bottle may be helpful.

If none of these remedies brings relief, you might try a pain reliever like aspirin or one of the nonaspirin pain relievers. Aspirin may be more effective than a nonaspirin pain reliever because aspirin is an antiprostaglandin, which means it acts against the prostaglandins. There are also aspirin-type medications made especially for menstrual pain. These medications usually contain some caffeine (the stimulant in coffee) as well. Sometimes this combination works where plain aspirin has failed.

If you've tried all these things and are still troubled by cramps, you should see a doctor. Severe cramps are sometimes a sign of some underlying medical problem. Also, a doctor can prescribe stronger pain relievers and antiprostaglandins than you can buy without a prescription.

If you do suffer from severe cramps, you may run into the "it's all in your head" attitude from the people around you, and from your doctor too. If so, try to ignore the people around you and find another doctor. It's very unlikely that your cramps are all in your head. Too many women have suffered too much needless

Exercise 1

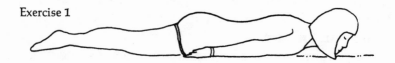

Gradually raise your head and chest without using your arms until your torso is off the floor.

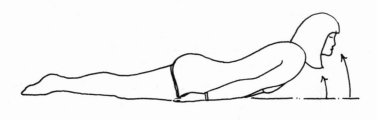

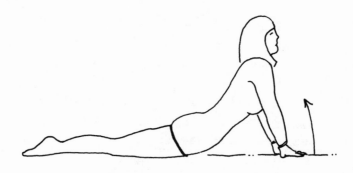

Using your arms, further raise your torso so that your back is arched. Repeat several times.

Illustration 36. Exercises for Menstrual Cramps

Exercise 2

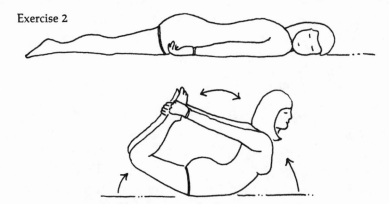

Begin by lying on your stomach. Grab your ankles with both hands, pulling forward toward the back of your head. Gently rock back and forth. Repeat several times.

Exercise 3

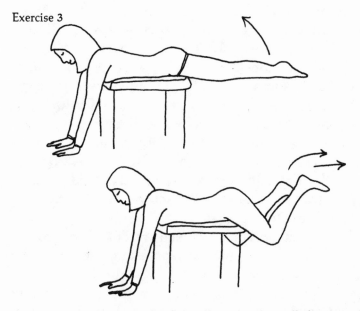

Lie on a coffee table or platform about 2–3 feet off the ground as shown here. Place your hands on the ground in front of you. Bend your knees and pull your ankles in toward your buttocks. Then in one smooth continuous motion, kick your legs out again. Continue until you gradually build up to do it for six minutes.

pain because of this "all in your head" business. If you have menstrual cramps, you deserve proper medical attention for your problem, so don't be afraid to insist upon it.

Menstrual Changes

Many women notice changes in their bodies or in their emotions that seem to take place during a certain phase of their menstrual cycle. For example, I get very energetic during my period and often get into fits of housecleaning (which is nice because, most of the time, I'm not too enthusiastic about housework). About a week and a half before my period starts, my breasts swell a bit and get very tender, or at times downright painful. (This only started happening since I turned thirty.) I often notice a change in my bowel movements during my period. Sometimes I get a slight touch of diarrhea; other times I'm constipated for a day or so. I sometimes have mild cramps or a full, pressured feeling in my lower abdomen while I'm menstruating. On the first couple of days of my period, I sometimes get what I call the "lead vagina" feeling. My vagina and vulva feel heavy, as if they were made of lead. (Well, it's not that bad, but "lead vagina" is a pretty good description.) I always know when I'm about to ovulate because I get to feeling very sexual.

Many of the girls and women we talked to also noticed emotional and physical changes that seemed to be related to their menstrual cycles. Most of these changes happen during their periods or in the week or so before their periods. These are some of the changes you may experience while you are menstruating or just before your period starts.

extra energy
lack of energy or a tired,
   dragged-out feeling
sudden shifts in moods
tension or anxiety
depression
feelings of wellbeing
bursts of creativity
a craving for sweets
pimples, acne, or other
   skin problems
a particularly clear and
   rosy glow to the skin
heightened sexual feelings
headaches
vision disturbances
diarrhea
constipation
swelling of the ankles,
   wrists, hands, or feet
swelling and tenderness
   of the breasts

swelling of the abdomen
bloated feeling
temporary weight gain
   (usually three to five
   pounds)
decreased ability to
   concentrate
increased ability to
   concentrate
increased appetite
increased thirst
cramps
increased need to urinate
urinary infections
a change in vaginal
   discharge
nausea
runny nose
sores in the mouth
backache

In some women, these changes are very noticeable; in others, they are hardly noticeable at all; and some women don't notice any changes in their bodies or their feelings over the course of their menstrual cycles.

Premenstrual Syndrome

Some women regularly experience one or two or more of the negative menstrual changes listed above during the seven to ten days preceding their menstrual period.

Such women are said to have premenstrual syndrome, or PMS. No one is sure what causes PMS. Some doctors think PMS is related to vitamin and nutritional deficiencies; others think that PMS is caused by a hormone imbalance.

Mild forms of PMS are quite widespread. As many as 40 percent of us experience some PMS symptoms at some time in our lives. It is not unusual, for example, for a woman to have a bloated feeling, pimples, swelling of the breasts, or other PMS symptoms in the week or so before her period.

If you have mild PMS symptoms, you may find that eliminating sugar, coffee, and chocolate from your diet, eating balanced meals with foods rich in vitamin B_6 and magnesium (green vegetables, whole grains, nuts, and seeds), and taking a vitamin supplement that includes the B complex vitamins will help alleviate symptoms. Some doctors use hormones to treat PMS, but others are not convinced that hormone treatments are really effective.

If you think you have PMS, you should consult a doctor familiar with the condition. For more information, write:

PMS Action
P.O. Box 9326
Madison, WI 53715

Optimox, Inc.
P.O. Box 7000-280
Palos Verdes Peninsula, CA 90074

Missing a Menstrual Period

If a woman gets pregnant, she stops having her menstrual period for the nine months that she is pregnant. She may start having her period again within a month or so after the baby is born, or it may take several months before she starts menstruating again. Women also miss periods as they are going through menopause. But menopause, pregnancy, and childbirth are not the only reasons why a woman sometimes misses periods. As we explained earlier, young women who've just started menstruating sometimes skip one or more periods on a regular basis. Even after a woman has been menstruating regularly for a number of years, she may occasionally skip one or more menstrual periods. This is quite normal and isn't anything to worry about; however, if you haven't had sexual intercourse with anyone and you miss three periods in a row, it's a good idea to see a doctor. Missing three periods in a row doesn't necessarily mean that there is something wrong with you. If you have had sexual intercourse and you miss a period, see you doctor *right away*, for you may be pregnant.

Not all women have menstrual periods every twenty-one to thirty-five days. Some women only have their periods once or twice a year; that's just the way their bodies work. But sometimes missing your periods is a sign that something is wrong. So, if you've missed three in a row, it's a good idea to see your doctor to determine whether you may have a medical problem that needs attention.

Other Menstrual Irregularities

There are also other menstrual irregularities that happen from time to time. As we explained earlier, some months your period may be heavier than others. This is quite normal, but sometimes the bleeding is excessive. If you are soaking through a pad or tampon (and we mean literally soaking through, so it's drenched with blood) every hour for an entire day, then it's a good idea to see your doctor.

Sometimes a woman's period doesn't stop. If your period continues for more than a week without showing any signs of slowing down or letting up, once again, you should see your doctor. If you've been having your period for seven days and you're still trickling out a bit of blood, that's nothing to worry about, but if the blood is still coming out as heavily as it was in the beginning of the week, you may have a problem.

Sometimes a woman's periods come too close together. As we explained earlier, traveling, illness, emotional ups and downs can all make your period come earlier or later than usual. But if three menstrual cycles go by where your cycle is less than eighteen days or more than thirty-five days apart, it's a good idea to see your doctor.

Some women experience what we call *spotting* between their periods. Spotting is a day or two of very light bleeding. It's not unusual for a woman to spot for a day or two around the time of ovulation. You can figure out whether your bleeding is related to ovulation by keeping track of your menstrual periods (see below) and noting the days when spotting occurs. Count back two weeks from the first day of bleeding of the next cycle. If the spotting occurs around two weeks before each period, it's probably related to ovulation and isn't anything to worry about. If the spotting occurs at other times and continues for more than three cycles, again, consult your doctor.

These are just guidelines to help you decide when to see your doctor about menstrual irregularities. If you feel there's something abnormal about your periods or if you are uncertain, don't hesitate to give your doctor a call and explain the problem. The two of you can then decide whether your problem warrants an office visit. Most menstrual irregularities are not serious, but sometimes they can indicate an underlying problem that needs attention, so don't hesitate to get any problems that are bothering you checked out.

Keeping Track of Your Menstrual Cycle

It's a good idea to keep a record of your menstrual cycles. That way, you'll learn how your own pattern works and will know about when to expect your next period. (Remember, though, that you may not be very regular at first.)

You'll need a calendar. On the first day of your period, that is, on the first day of bleeding, mark an *x* on your calendar. Continue to mark an *x* for as long as the bleeding continues. When your next period starts, mark an *x* again. You might want to count the number of days between your periods and note that figure so you'll begin to get an idea of how long your menstrual cycle usually lasts (see Illustration 37).

S	M	T	W	Th	F	S
		1	2	3	4	5
6	7	8	9̸	1̸0̸	1̸1̸	1̸2̸
1̸3̸	1̸4̸	15	16	17	18	19
20	21	22	23	24	25	26
27	28	29	30			

S	M	T	W	Th	F	S
				1	2	3
4	5	6	7	8̸	9̸	1̸0̸
1̸1̸	1̸2̸	13	14	15	16	17
18	19	20	21	22	23	24
25	26	27	28	29	30	

Illustration 37. Recording Your Periods. To keep track of your periods, use a calendar like this. This girl had her first day of bleeding on the ninth and she continued to bleed for five more days, so she marked these days with x's. The next cycle began on the eighth of the following month and her period lasted 5 days, which are marked with x's. By counting the number of days between x's, you can determine the length of your period. This girl's cycle was 28 days long.

You might also want to make a note of cramps, ovulation pain, or any of the other menstrual changes you may notice. If, for instance, you find that you have a craving for sweets, that you feel tense and cranky, or that your breasts are tender, note this on your calendar, so that you can begin to learn about your body's patterns.

CHAPTER 8

Puberty in Boys

This book was written for girls, to help them understand how puberty happens in their bodies. But puberty doesn't just happen to girls; it happens to boys, too. Since most girls are curious about boys' bodies, we decided to include a brief chapter on how puberty happens in boys (see Illustration 38).

In some ways, puberty in boys is similar to puberty in girls. In both sexes, there is a sudden growth spurt and a change in the general shape of the body. Both boys and girls begin to grow pubic hair and other body hair. Girls produce ripe ova for the first time, and boys begin to make sperm, the male counterpart of ova. The genital organs of both sexes begin to develop and grow larger. Both boys and girls begin to perspire more and tend to get pimples at this time in their lives.

But boys and girls are different, so puberty is a bit different in boys than it is in girls. For one thing,

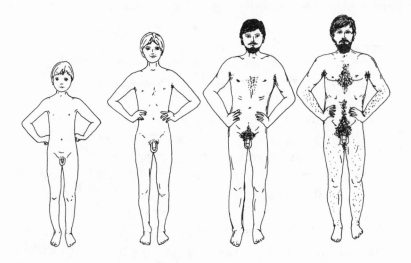

Illustration 38. Boys in Puberty. Like girls, boys too go through puberty. They get taller, their shoulders get wider, their bodies more muscular, their genital organs develop, and they begin to grow hair on their chests, arms, legs genitals, underarms, and faces.

puberty usually happens earlier in girls. The average girl starts puberty about two years before the average boy. But as we have seen, not everyone is average. Some girls start earlier than average, some later. The same is true of boys; some boys will actually start puberty before some of the girls their age.

Because boys and girls are different, some of the things that happen in a girl's body during puberty don't happen to boys and vice versa. Obviously, boys don't start having menstrual periods. And other things that happen to boys, such as a deepening and a lowering of the voice, don't happen to girls.

Circumcision

Illustration 1 on page 23 shows the sex organs on the outside of a man's body. You might want to take another look at that picture before reading this chapter so that you'll remember the names of the various parts of the male genitals.

Illustration 1 shows a penis that has been *circumcised*. *Circumcision* is an operation in which the foreskin, a sheath of skin that covers the glans, is cut away. Circumcision is usually done shortly after a boy is born, but it may also be done when a boy is older. Not all males are circumcised. If a boy or man has not been circumcised, the foreskin covers the glans. As you can see in Illustration 39, the foreskin is loose and can be stretched out or slid down the shaft of the penis so that the glans is exposed.

Sometimes, a boy is circumcised for religious reasons. Some Jewish and Moslem parents have their boy babies circumcised because it is a custom in their

circumcision (sir-come-SISH-un)
circumcised (sir-come-SIZED)

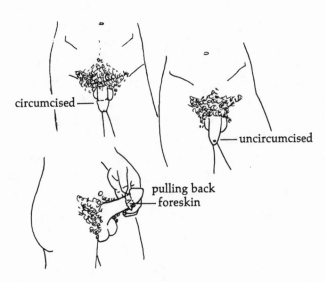

Illustration 39. Circumcised and Uncircumcised Penis

religion. Until recently, most boys in this country were circumcised even if their parents weren't Jewish or Moslem. Doctors encouraged parents to have their babies circumcised because it was thought that men who weren't circumcised were more likely to get cancer of the penis than men who had been circumcised. Doctors are no longer certain that being circumcised really has anything to do with how likely it is that a man will get cancer of the penis. Moreover, cancer of the penis is a rare disease. So, nowadays, a lot of parents are wondering whether it's really worthwhile to put a newborn baby through the pain of circumcision. More and more parents are deciding not to have their male babies circumcised.

The only difference between circumcised and uncircumcised males is that circumcised males don't have a foreskin; otherwise, their penises look, feel, and work the same way.

The Penis and Scrotum

The penis is made up of spongy tissue. There is a hollow tube called the *urethra* that runs down the inside of the penis. When a male urinates, the urine passes through this tube and comes out the opening at the tip of the glans. Sperm travel through this same tube and come out at this same opening when a man ejaculates (a valve on the bladder prevents sperm and urine from coming out at the same time).

Underneath the penis lies the scrotum, the skin sac that holds the two testicles. The testicles are very sensitive and it can be very painful if they are hit or knocked about.

Five Stages of Genital Development

The appearance of a boy's penis and scrotum changes as he goes through puberty. During childhood, a boy's scrotum is drawn up close to his body. As he goes through puberty, the scrotum begins to get looser and to hang down. When a man or boy is cold or frightened or feeling sexual, his scrotum may get tighter and draw up close to his body for a while. The penis and scrotum also get larger as a boy goes through puberty and pubic hair begins to grow around the genitals.

Just as doctors have divided the breast and pubic hair development of girls into five separate stages, so they have divided the growth of male genital organs into five stages (see Illustration 40).

Stage 1 starts at birth and continues until the boy starts Stage 2. The penis, scrotum, and testicles don't change very much during this stage, but there is a slight increase in overall size.

In Stage 2, the testicles start to grow and to hang down more. One testis may hang lower than the other. The skin of the scrotum darkens in color and gets rougher in texture. The penis gets somewhat larger.

During Stage 3, the penis gets longer and somewhat wider. The testes and scrotum continue to get larger, and the skin of the penis and scrotum may continue to get darker.

By Stage 4, the penis has gotten considerably longer and wider. The testes and scrotum have also gotten larger, and the skin of the penis and scrotum may still be getting darker.

Stage 5 is the adult stage in which the penis has reached its full width and length, and the testicles and scrotum are fully developed.

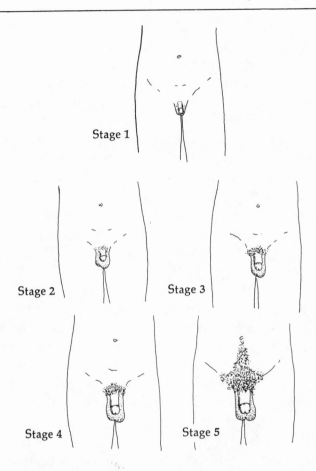

Illustration 40. The Five Stages of Male Genital Development

A boy's genitals may start developing when he is as young as nine years of age, but some boys don't start until they are fifteen or older. The average boy starts puberty after his eleventh or twelfth birthday. But, of course, not all boys are average, so some start earlier and others later. Most boys take about three or four years to go from Stage 2 to Stage 5, but some boys take less than two years, and others take five or more years.

Starting early or starting late doesn't have any effect on how long it takes a boy to go through these stages. Some early starters develop quickly, others grow slowly. The same is true for late starters: Some grow quickly, others slowly. Starting early or starting late doesn't have anything to do with how large a boy's penis will be when he's fully grown. Late starters may end up with either large or small penises, and the same goes for early starters. Just as breast size doesn't have anything to do with how feminine or womanly a female is, so penis size doesn't have anything to do with how masculine a male is.

Pubic Hair and Other Body Hair

Boys also start to grow pubic hair as they go through puberty. Boy's pubic hair is similar to girl's pubic hair. At first, there are only a few, slightly curly hairs, but as puberty continues, the hairs get curlier and darker in color, and there are more of them. The pubic hair first starts to grow around the base of the penis. Then, a few hairs begin to grow on the scrotum. As a boy gets older, pubic hair starts to grow on his lower belly and up toward his belly button. It may also grow down around his anus. It may start growing out onto his thighs. The pubic hairs usually don't start to grow until after the testes have started developing.

Boys also start to grow hair in their armpits during puberty. This usually happens about a year or so after the pubic hair has started growing, but some boys start growing hair under their arms before they have any pubic hair.

During puberty, boys also grow hair on their faces. The hair usually starts growing on the corners of the upper lips. Sideburns may start to grow at the same time. The moustache continues to grow, and then hair grows on the upper part of the cheek and just below the middle of the lower lip. Finally, it grows on the chin. Hair doesn't usually start growing on the chin until a boy's genitals are fully developed. For most boys, facial hair starts growing between the ages of fourteen and eighteen, but it may start earlier or later.

The hair on a boy's arms and legs tends to get darker and thicker during puberty. Some boys grow hair on their chests and back too. Some develop quite a bit of hair on their chests; others have very little.

Changing Shape and Size

Girls' bodies get curvier during puberty and boys' bodies get more muscular. Their shoulders get broader and their arms and legs get thicker. Boys also have a growth spurt during puberty. Their growth spurt is more dramatic than girls'. It lasts longer, and boys grow taller than girls on average. It usually happens about two years later than girls' growth spurt. Generally, it doesn't happen until their penises have started to grow.

Skin Changes

Like girls', boys' skin also begins to change during puberty. The oil glands become more active, and most boys develop some pimples. Boys, too, begin to perspire more heavily during puberty and their perspiration may have a different odor. Like girls, some boys develop purplish marks on the skin that usually appear on the hips and buttocks. As they grow older, these marks fade.

Breasts

Boys' breasts don't, of course, go through the same kind of changes that girls' do during puberty, but a boy's areola does get wider during puberty. Most boys' breasts swell a bit during puberty and, like girls, boys sometimes notice a feeling of tenderness or soreness in their breasts at this time. This swelling usually starts during Stage 2 or 3. It may happen to both breasts or only to one. It may only last a few months or a year, but it may continue for two years or even longer. Eventually, though, it goes away.

Voice

Boys' voices change during puberty, getting lower and deeper. While their voices are changing, some boys' voices have a tendency to "crack," to shift suddenly from a low pitch to a high, squeaky pitch. This cracking may only last for a few months, but sometimes it goes on for a year or two.

Erections

Way back in Chapter 1, on page 28, we talked about erections. When a man or a boy has an erection, blood rushes to the penis and fills up the spongy tissues inside the penis. Muscles at the base of the penis tighten up so the blood stays in the penis for a while, making it feel hard. During an erection, the penis gets longer and wider and, usually, darker in color, and it stands erect, away from the body as in Illustration 41.

Males get erections throughout their lives, even when they are tiny babies. Stroking or touching the penis or scrotum can cause an erection. Getting sexually excited and having sexual fantasies can cause an erection. Males can also get erections even if the penis and scrotum aren't being touched or rubbed and even if they aren't feeling or thinking about anything sexual. Some males wake up in the morning with erections. Having to urinate will cause erections sometimes.

During puberty, boys are apt to get erections more frequently. As they go through puberty, most boys start to experience what we call "spontaneous erections." Spontaneous erections are erections that happen all by themselves, without the penis or scrotum being touched or rubbed.

Spontaneous erections can be very embarrassing for a boy. They may happen when he is in school, at home, walking down the street, or just about any time or place. It's a popular myth in our society that girls are much more embarrassed by the changes that happen in their bodies during puberty—growing breasts, having their periods, and so on—than boys. But the boys in

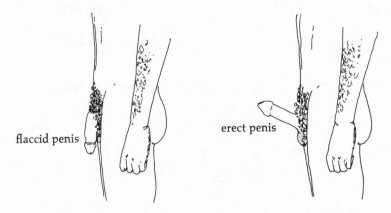

flaccid penis

erect penis

Illustration 41. Flaccid and Erect Penis. When a man or boy has an erection the soft, spongy tissue inside the penis fills with blood. The penis gets stiff and hard and stands out from his body.

my classes had a lot of stories to tell about getting spontaneous erections and worrying that the people around them would notice the bulge in their pants from the erection.

When a male has an erection, one of two things may happen. The erection may go away all by itself. The muscles at the base of the penis may relax, allowing the blood to leave the penis, so that it gets smaller and soft again. Or he may masturbate or have sexual intercourse until he has an orgasm. During an orgasm, the muscles of the penis release and contract rhythmically, and shortly after the orgasm, the muscles at the base of the penis relax, allowing the blood to leave and the penis to get soft again.

Sperm and Ejaculation

Like girls, boys begin to make their first ripe seeds, the sperm, during puberty. The cross section in Illustration 42 shows the inside of the penis and scrotum. The sperm are made inside tiny little tubes that are coiled

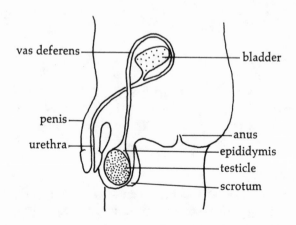

Illustration 42. Cross-Section of the Penis, Scrotum, and Testicle

up inside the testicle. They then travel through these tubes to the *epididymis*, which is a sort of storage area or compartment. The sperm spend about six weeks in the epididymis where they finish ripening. They travel from the epididymis through a tube called the *vas deferens* to another set of storage compartments located outside the testicle. These storage compartments (not shown) are called *seminal vesicles*.

In order to get from the seminal vesicles to the outside of the body, the sperm must travel through the urethra, the tube in the center of the penis. Urine from the bladder also travels down this tube, but urine and sperm can't travel through the urethra at the same time. There is a little valve on the bladder that closes off the bladder any time the sperm are about to come out.

As we explained in Chapter 1, on pages 29-30, when a man ejaculates, the muscles of the erect penis contract and force the sperm up this tube and out the opening in the end of the penis. Just as having her first menstrual period is a landmark for girls going through puberty, so having the first ejaculation is a landmark for boys.

A boy may have his first ejaculation while he is masturbating. Many of the boys in our class had their first ejaculations in this way. Others have their first ejaculation in their sleep. This is known as having a wet dream. The boy wakes up and finds one or two table-spoonfuls of creamy, white liquid on his belly or his bedclothes. If he hasn't been prepared for it, having a wet dream can come as quite a surprise.

epididymis (eh-pih-DIH-dih-miss)
vas (VAS)
deferens (DEAF-eh-renz)
seminal (SEM-in-ul)
vesicles (VES-eh-kuls)

Wet dreams are the male body's way of relieving the testicles of a buildup of sperm. If a boy masturbates a lot during the day, then he may not have wet dreams at night, for masturbating until he ejaculates will also empty out the buildup of sperm in the testicles.

As you can see, boys, as well as girls, go through puberty. Their bodies change and they too are getting ready for the time in their lives when they may decide to have babies.

CHAPTER 9

Sexuality

> If a girl is thirteen and she's had her period and all she
> ever thinks about is boys and sex, is this normal?

This question came out of our "Everything You Ever
Wanted to Know" question box. Questions like this
come up all the time in our puberty classes because, as
we go through puberty, many of us experience stronger
sexual feelings than ever before in our lives. For some,
this means the urge to masturbate more often or to
spend more time having sexual fantasies. For others, it
means having very strong sexual and romantic attractions to someone or spending more time having fantasies in which they imagine a passionate romance with
a special someone. These sexual and romantic feelings
can be very intense and distracting. It may seem as if
sex and romance are all you can think about. Some
girls get so preoccupied that it's a bit scary for them. It

helps to know that these feelings are perfectly normal and that a lot of other people your age are going through the same thing.

Not everyone experiences intense romantic or sexual feelings during puberty. Some get involved in school, sports, music, a job, or another aspect of their lives, and sex and romance just aren't major interests for them. But since the body changes of puberty often *do* spark an interest in sex and romance, many young people are curious about these things.

In the following pages we'll be talking about sexuality. Sexuality means many things. People tend to think that sexuality refers just to having sexual intercourse, but it encompasses much more. Masturbation, kissing, touching yourself or someone else in a sexual way, being attracted to another person, being in love, having romantic or sexual feelings or fantasies—all these things are part of our sexuality. It would take an entire book (or maybe several books) to discuss sexuality thoroughly. So, in this chapter, we're just going to mention certain aspects of sexuality, concentrating on some of the sexual problems and issues that may come up as you move through puberty and into your teen years. We'll also suggest other books in the section "For Further Reading" that follows this chapter and other sources of information that might prove helpful.

Crushes

Many girls (and boys, too) develop crushes as they go through puberty. Having a crush can be very exciting. Just catching a glimpse of the person you have a crush on can brighten your whole day, and you may spend delightful hours imagining a romance with that person.

Crushes can also be a safe and healthy way of experimenting with romantic and sexual attractions.

Sometimes young people develop crushes on someone who isn't very likely to return their affections—on a movie star, a rock singer, or a teacher at school. And that's just fine, but having a crush on someone unattainable can also cause a lot of suffering. One year some of the girls in my class developed crushes on a certain rock star. They plastered their bedroom walls with posters, sported buttons with his face printed on them, pored over fan magazines, and generally had a great time sharing their feelings about him with one another. When the rock star got married, they were, naturally, somewhat disappointed, but one girl was more than disappointed. She was really upset. She had gotten too involved in her crush, and the rock star's marriage was devastating for her. If you find yourself developing a serious crush on someone unattainable, it helps to remind yourself from time to time that your crush isn't very realistic and that this person isn't very likely to return your affections.

Not all crushes are unrealistic. You may develop a crush on someone near your own age whom you actually know through school or church or some other group. If that person is interested in you, the crush can be especially exciting. But even with someone you know, yearning after a person who doesn't return your affections can be painful. If you find that your crushes or your sexual feelings are causing you problems, it helps to find someone—a friend, a parent, a teacher, another adult, or a counselor—to talk things over with.

For most of us, our first crushes are very special, and as long as we don't lose our perspective, they can be a wonderful and positive part of growing up.

Dating

As you move through puberty and into the teen years, many girls begin dating. Dating can be fun and exciting, but it can also create problems. You may want to date before your parents think you're old enough. Or you may not be ready to date, and your parents may be pushing you into it. You may have trouble deciding whether you want to go steady with one person or date lots of different people. If you've been dating one person steadily and decide you want to go out with others, you may have problems ending your steady dating relationship. Or if your steady decides to change the relationship with you, you may have a hard time dealing with this. On the other hand, if you want to date and no one is asking you out, you may get to feeling rather blue.

Some of the best advice we've come across on dating and how to handle these and other problems is contained in books described in the section "For Further Reading."

Making Decisions About Sex

Once you begin dating, you may find yourself having to make decisions about how you want to handle your sexuality. Is it all right to kiss on your first date? What about french kissing (putting your tongue in someone's mouth as you're kissing)? Is necking or making out (spending time kissing and hugging) okay? What about moving beyond making out and into petting "above the waist" (touching a girl's breasts) or "below the waist" (touching and rubbing the other person's genitals)? How about oral sex (using your mouth and tongue to stimulate the other person's sex organs)? What about sexual intercourse? When is it okay to have these kinds of sexual experiences and when is it not okay?

Some young people feel very clear about these issues. They know exactly how far they want to go. For example, some people feel that anything more than making out, or perhaps petting, is not okay, and that people shouldn't have sexual intercourse until after they're married. Others are not so certain. They might, for instance, feel that sexual intercourse is okay if the people are old enough and are really in love. But what's "old enough" and how do you know if you're really in love?

In the end, only you can answer these questions or make your decisions about how to handle sexuality, but you can get some help. You can start by talking these issues over with other people. Older people who've had some sexual experience can be helpful. What do they think, and why do they feel the way they do? Don't (as many young people do) automatically rule out your parents as people to talk to. Young people often don't talk about sexual decision-making with their parents because they already know that their parents' attitudes are more conservative or stricter than theirs. But even if this is so, your parents may have good reasons for feeling the way they do. And even if you don't totally agree with them, they might have things to say that could prove useful to your life. You might also talk with other older people—an aunt or uncle, a sister or brother, a counselor or older teens.

You might want to join a "rap" group where you can meet with other people your own age to talk about sexual decision-making and other problems that young people face. In some cities, Planned Parenthood has rap groups for young people. These groups are run by peer counselors, teen-agers who've been well educated about sexuality and who are experienced in leading group discussions. A community hotline, a women's center or health-care clinic, the YWCA might also be able to put you in touch with a teen group in your area.

There is often tremendous pressure on young people to experiment sexually. If you are having a relationship with someone, that person may be pressuring you to go further than you really feel ready to. Someone may be insisting that you "prove that you really love me," or the other person may threaten to stop seeing you if you don't go along. It might be helpful for you to know how other teen-agers feel about these pressures. Talk to your friends or have a look at some of the books described in "For Further Reading."

Birth Control

If you do decide to have sexual intercourse, you need to use some form of birth control if you don't want to get pregnant. Some young people believe that you can't get pregnant the first time you have sexual intercourse. This is *not true*. It is perfectly possible, and there are many, many women who have gotten pregnant the first time they had sex. Others who have been having sex for a while without getting pregnant develop a false sense of confidence. They figure that since they've gotten away with it so far, they'll continue to get away with it. This is also *not true*. In fact, the longer a woman continues to have sexual intercourse without using birth control, the greater her chances of getting pregnant. Some young people think, "It can't happen to me," that pregnancy is something that only happens to other people. Again, *not true*. Any woman who has sexual intercourse without using birth control may get pregnant, and most of them do sooner or later.

While we're on the subject of things that are not true, it is also not true that you can't get pregnant if you jump up and down after you have sex to shake the sperm out of you. It is not true that a woman can't get pregnant if she has sex while she's having her menstrual period. It is not true that douching after sex will prevent pregnancy. And it is not true that a woman can't get pregnant if a man pulls his penis out of her vagina before he ejaculates. When a man's penis gets erect, he produces a few drops of fluid from the end of his penis. This fluid may contain sperm. So even if a man pulls out his penis before he comes, he may still leave some sperm in the vagina. Also, if he ejaculates near the opening to the vagina, the sperm may still be able to swim up into the vagina.

Even if you're not having sexual intercourse yet, it's a good idea to learn about birth control. There are many different methods of birth control. Some are permanent methods, but most are only temporary. Some methods have side effects and are more dangerous to use than other methods. Some methods are easier or more convenient to use than others. Some methods require a doctor's prescription; others don't. It's important to become well informed so that you can eventually choose what is best for you. Fortunately, there are any number of excellent books that deal with birth control. Some are listed in "For Further Reading." Planned Parenthood clinics in some cities offer special classes on birth control for teens.

Sexually Transmitted Diseases

If you decide to have sexual intercourse, you also need to know about sexually transmitted diseases. Sexually transmitted diseases, which are also called *STDs*, *venereal diseases*, or *VD*, are infections that are usually transmitted from one person to another through sexual contact. There are a number of different kinds of STDs. The most common ones are gonorrhea, or "clap," syphillis, and herpes. Gonorrhea and syphillis can be cured, but if they are not treated promptly, they can cause serious illness. There is no cure for herpes. Herpes is more serious as there is no known cure. It has caused birth defects in the babies of some of the women who have it and can increase a woman's chance of getting a certain type of cancer. Herpes is a very common disease and one about which you should be well informed. To find out more about herpes, write to H.E.L.P., Box 100, Palo Alto, CA 94302.

Because STDs are transmitted through sexual activity, people are often embarrassed to seek treatment or to tell their sex partners that they may have given them an STD. It's important for you to learn the signs and symptoms of STDs, how to avoid getting an STD, and what to do if you get one. (See "For Further Reading" for some books that deal with STDs.) If you think you may have contracted an STD, you can get information and help in getting treatment by calling the National VD Hotline. In all states except California, call 1-800-227-8922. In California, call 1-800-982-5883. Because these are 800 numbers, there is no charge for the call, and if you call from your home telephone the charge will not appear on your bill. The call is private and confidential. You don't have to tell them your name.

Homosexual Feelings

We use the word *homosexual* to describe sexual or romantic feelings or sexual activities that involve people of the same sex. Having a crush on another girl or on a woman (or for a boy, on another male) can be very scary and confusing because, in our culture, we are usually taught to think that the only "right" or acceptable sexual or romantic feelings are those that center around someone of the opposite sex. People make jokes about homosexuals and use derogatory terms such as "queer," "fairy," or "fag" for male homosexuals and "butch," "dyke," or "bulldyke" for female homosexuals. As a result, most of us have a great fear of homosexuality.

But psychologists who study sexuality have found that the vast majority of us have homosexual feelings, fantasies, dreams, or actual homosexual experiences at some time. These don't make you homosexual. If you have homosexual feelings or experiences, you're apt to feel a bit uncomfortable about it. It helps to know the facts.

About one in ten people in this country is homosexual, which means mainly attracted to people of the same sex. Female homosexuals are also called lesbians, and the word *gays* is used to refer to both male and female homosexuals.

Some gay people are exclusively homosexual. Throughout their lives, all their sexual attractions, dreams, fantasies, and sexual activities involve people of the same sex as they are. But most gay people are not exclusively homosexual. At some time in their lives they have feelings, fantasies, or experiences that involve people of the opposite sex.

Heterosexuals (people whose sexual feelings, fantasies, and/or experiences are with people of the opposite sex) may also have homosexual feelings, fantasies, or sexual experiences at times. People often think that if they have homosexual fantasies or even just one homosexual experience, this means that they are homosexuals. This is not true.

If you have homosexual thoughts, feelings, or homosexual experiences at times, it helps to know that this is natural and normal. If you're pretty sure that you're "more gay" than not, it helps to know that this too is natural and that you're not alone. If you're interested in learning more about homosexuality, there are some books listed in "For Further Reading" following this chapter that you will find helpful.

Rape

Another sexual matter that comes up for some young people is rape. *Rape* means being forced to have sex against your will. It can happen to anyone, at any age. If it happens to you, it's important that you know what to do.

The most important thing to do is get help right away. Some girls (and women, too) are so upset by what has happened to them that they just want to go home and try to forget about it. You need *immediate* medical attention. Even if you don't seem to have any serious injuries, you could have internal injuries that need treatment. You will also need a test to make sure you haven't gotten pregnant as a result of the rape. (If the doctor thinks it likely that the rape has resulted in a pregnancy, there are pills that can protect you from a pregnancy. These pills, which are more effective the sooner they are taken, carry some risks, but in the case of rape, you may decide to take the risk.) You will also need tests to determine whether you have gotten a sexually transmitted disease as a result of the rape.

(These tests are one reason why you shouldn't bathe or shower before seeing the doctor.) And you should seek help because you will need support to help you recover emotionally, as well as physically.

Depending upon the circumstances of the rape, there are a number of ways to go about getting help. You can go to a hospital emergency room or call the police, who will take you to the hospital. Many communities have rape crisis centers or rape hotlines (listed under "Rape" in the telephone book). If you can get in touch with a rape center or hotline, do so. The people there are specially trained. They can tell you which hospitals in your area have the best programs for aiding rape victims and can often send someone to get you and take you to the hospital.

Rape is a very common crime, and it's important to be informed in case it happens to you or to someone you know.

Incest

Rape is a very serious and scary matter. Incest can be equally upsetting and shocking. Incest involves a family member being sexual with another family member. This may be anything from touching, feeling, or kissing sexual organs to actual sexual intercourse. It often happens with brothers and sisters as they are growing up. Incest between brothers and sisters is not always a harmful or upsetting thing. In fact, many brothers and sisters engage in some form of sex play as children. But being pressured or forced into having sexual contact with an older relative can be harmful.

Incest can happen to very young children and to

teen-agers. Most victims of incest are girls who are victimized by a father, stepfather, uncle—indeed, by any male family member. Sometimes boys are victims of incest by a male relative, too. Incest between boys and their older female relatives is rare.

Incest isn't necessarily a forced thing like rape. Because of the older person's position in the family, he may be able to pressure a girl into doing things without having to force her physically.

Some incest victims feel it's their fault because they enjoyed some aspect of the incest. Incest sometimes starts at a very early age, and only when the girl gets older does she realize that these sexual activities are somewhat strange and unsettling.

Most incest victims feel a mixture of guilt, shame, humiliation, and anger. If you are a victim of incest, there's really only one thing to do: *Tell someone.* Telling someone can be very hard. First of all, you may not be believed. For example, many mothers refuse to believe their daughters at first. If your mom won't believe you, try finding someone else, an aunt, a grandmother, an older sister or brother, a teacher or any adult who you feel will believe you. You can also call a local rape crisis center or hotline, Planned Parenthood, a woman's center, the YWCA, or a community mental-health center.

Another thing that makes it difficult to tell someone is that incest is a crime. But most people who commit incest aren't sent to jail. Usually, the judge sends the person for some sort of psychiatric treatment. People who commit incest are sick, but they can be cured. The person who commits incest needs help, and the victim and other family members also need help.

A Few Final Words

You're growing up, and growing up isn't always an easy thing to do. In this chapter, we've concentrated on some very serious topics—rape, incest, STDs, birth control, and so forth. It's important to know about these things, but it's also important to remember that growing up has its more positive sides. We are becoming sexual beings as we move through puberty and into adulthood. Sexuality is a rich and meaningful part of our lives, a source of deep joy and contentment, and puberty, despite the problems it may present, is an exciting time in our lives. It is a time of many "firsts"—first period, first date, first kiss, first love, first job, first driver's license. It is a time when we begin to become our very own independent selves. We hope that this book has helped you to understand more about your puberty and to enjoy it all the more.

FOR FURTHER READING

AUSTIN, AL and HEFNER, KEITH, eds. *Growing Up Gay* (Ann Arbor: Youth Liberation Press, 1978).

This collection of essays, written by gay young people, deals with the issues homosexuals face as they are growing up. To order, send $1.75 to Youth Liberation Press, 2007 Washington Avenue, Ann Arbor, Michigan 48104.

BELL, RUTH. *Changing Bodies, Changing Lives: A Book for Teens on Sex and Relationships* (New York: Random House, 1981).

Absolutely the best book for teens on the topic, representing many points of view through quotes from teenagers themselves. The first section deals with the physical changes of puberty, including how it feels to have a wet dream, a first period, etc. The next section deals with interpersonal issues between parents and teens and teens and peers, as well as loneliness, love, marriage, divorce, and sex role expectations. The middle two sections of the book are devoted to sexuality and cover masturbation, sexual fantasies, kissing, petting, making decisions about how far to go, saying no, homosexuality, oral-genital sex, intercourse, and sexual problems, without taking a specific stand on moral issues. There is also an excellent section on rape and incest and good information on drugs and alcohol, sexually transmitted diseases, and birth control. The section on teenage pregnancy is especially good, and the one on mental health, depression, and suicide is outstanding. The book is geared toward the fourteen- to nineteen-year-old age group but could be valuable for younger and older people as well.

BLUME, JUDY. *Deenie* (New York: Dell, 1974).

Thirteen-year-old Deenie is being pushed into a modeling career by her mother, but Deenie herself is more interested in spending time with her girl friends, going to the school dance to hear Buddy play his drums, and tracking Harvey Grabowsky, the captain of the football team, through Woolworth's. The novel presents a portrait of a young girl's life that preteens and young teens can identify with and touches on such topics as masturbation and sexual intercourse. This is just one of Blume's many fine books for preteens and teens.

COMFORT, ALEX and JANE. *The Facts of Love: Living, Loving, and Growing* (New York: Crown, 1979).

Although it can't compare to Ruth Bell's *Changing Bodies, Changing Lives,* this book covers many of the same topics in a comprehensive and straightforward manner. It could serve as a nice bridge between this book and *Changing Bodies* and is especially good for younger adolescents (ages ten to thirteen). The illustrations are lovely. More conservative parents may be more comfortable with this book than with the much franker presentation in *Changing Bodies;* however, in my experience, teens themselves much prefer Bell's book. Parents who worry that presenting information about sexuality to their children might lead to promiscuous behavior owe it to themselves to read the introduction to *The Facts of Love.*

THE DIAGRAM GROUP. *Sex: A User's Manual* (New York: Berkeley, 1982).

This is an extremely straightforward, up-to-date guide that covers virtually every aspect of sexual experience, sexual development, and social attitudes about sex, including methods of intercourse, the phases of sexual excitement, foreplay, orgasm, unconventional sex practices, sexual problems, sex crimes, and prostitution. It also discusses attraction and courtship, birth control, and sexually transmitted diseases. The book is aimed at an adult audience, but the information is presented in a well-illustrated format and is written in clear, simple prose that teens can readily understand. Again, more conservative parents may feel uncomfortable with this book because it deals so openly with the varieties of sexual behavior.

EAGAN, ANDREA BOROFF. *Why Am I So Miserable If These Are the Best Years of My Life?* (New York: Avon, 1979).

Although the information on birth control and sexually transmitted diseases in this book is a bit out of date, it is still valuable for its advice to teenage girls on dealing with conflicts between parents and daughters, dating, going steady, friendships with other girls, restrictive sex roles, the double standard, making decisions about sex, saying no, being part of the "in" group, and feelings of loneliness. It has an especially good discussion about the boy-does-the-asking tradition in dating and the risks and rewards for girls who try to take the initiative.

GARDNER-LOULAN, JOANN; LOPEZ, BONNIE; and QUACKENBUSH, MARIA. *Period* (San Francisco: Volcano Press, 1981).

This excellent picture book deals with menstruation and is especially useful for introducing preteens to the topic. The illustrations, which feature all ethnic groups and even handicapped kids (which most books don't do), are marvelous and depict all types of girls, not just conventionally pretty, idealized body types.

MADARAS, LYNDA and PATTERSON, JANE. *Womancare: A Gynecological Guide to Your Body.* (New York: Avon Books, 1981).

Although I may be a bit prejudiced about this one (since I am one of the authors), I think it is an excellent guide to medical problems and birth control. It was written for an adult audience but covers birth control, sexually transmitted diseases, vaginal infections, menstrual problems, toxic shock syndrome, and other medical problems that may affect young women.

MIKLOWITZ, GLORIA D. *Did You Hear What Happened to Andrea?* (New York: Delacorte, 1979).

This novel tells the story of Andrea, a fifteen-year-old girl who is raped. It not only discusses rape, but it also deals with the difficulties Andrea has afterward with her parents, friends, and boyfriends. It is an invaluable book for any young person who has undergone the trauma of rape, or, for that matter, for any young person. Like Judy Blume, the author has also written other exceptional books for preteens and teenagers.

SILVERSTEIN, CHARLES. *A Family Matter: A Parent's Guide to Homosexuality* (New York: McGraw-Hill, 1978).

Although this book was written for parents rather than young people themselves, it's an excellent book and helpful for both adults and young people.

STEWART, FELICIA; GUEST, FELICIA; STEWART, GARY; and HATCHER, ROBERT. *My Body, My Health.* (New York: John Wiley, 1979).

This book was written for adult women, but the language is simple enough for younger women too. It is an excellent source of information on birth control, sexually transmitted diseases, vaginal infections and other medical problems. It also has an informative chapter on rape and another on sexual problems.

Index

ABOUT THE AUTHORS

Lynda Madaras is the author of *Child's Play* and co-author of *Womancare, Great Expectations,* and *The Alphabet Connection.* She lectures frequently on women's healthcare subjects and teaches classes in puberty and sex education to teens and pre-teens. When considering how to have "the talk" with her own daughter, she became aware of just how few books there are she could share with her. She designed this book for mother and daughter to read together.

Area Madaras assisted her mother in the book's preparation.